Mediterranean Diet Meal Prep:

Delicious and Healthy Recipes of The Mediterranean Diet. Reduce Weight, Saving Time and Feeling at your Absolute Best with The Mediterranean Diet

BY

SARAH COOPERS

indirect, which are incurred as a result of the use of information contained within this document, including, but not limited to, — errors, omissions, or inaccuracies.

Table of Contents

INTRODUCTION

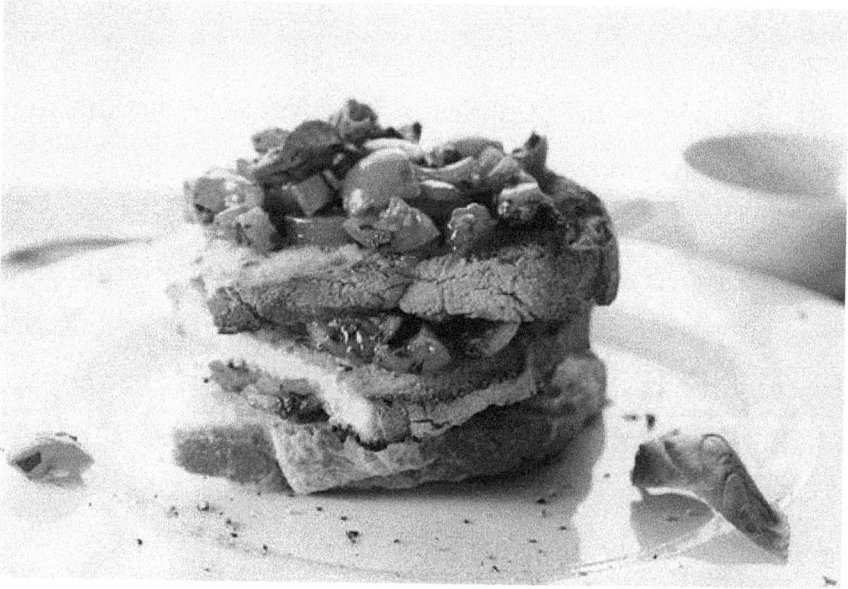

In case you're searching for a heart-good dieting arrangement, the Mediterranean eating regimen may be directly for you. The Mediterranean eating routine mixes the fundamentals of smart dieting with the customary flavors and cooking techniques for the Mediterranean.

Why the Mediterranean eating routine?

Enthusiasm for the Mediterranean eating regimen started during the 1960s with the perception that coronary illness caused fewer passing in Mediterranean nations, for example, Greece and Italy than in the U.S. what's more, northern Europe. Ensuing studies found that the Mediterranean diet is related to diminished hazard factors for the cardiovascular malady. The Mediterranean eating regimen is one of the excellent dieting plans prescribed by the Dietary Guidelines for Americans to advance wellbeing and forestall constant infection.

It is likewise perceived by the World Health Organization as a sound and reasonable dietary example and as an immaterial social resource by the United National Educational, Scientific, and Cultural Organization.

What is the Mediterranean eating routine?

The Mediterranean eating routine is a method for eating dependent on the customary cooking of nations circumscribing the Mediterranean Sea. While there is no single meaning of the Mediterranean eating routine, it usually is high in vegetables, organic products, entire grains, beans, nut and seeds, and olive oil.

The fundamental segments of Mediterranean eating regimen include:

• Daily utilization of vegetables, organic products, entire grains, and solid fats

• Weekly admission of fish, poultry, beans, and eggs

• Moderate parts of dairy items

• Limited admission of red meat

Other significant components of the Mediterranean diet are offering suppers to loved ones, getting a charge out of a glass of red wine, and being physically dynamic.

Plant-based, not meat-based

The establishment of the Mediterranean eating regimen is vegetables, organic products, herbs, nuts, beans, and entire grains. Dinners are worked around these plant-based nourishments. Moderate measures of dairy, poultry, and eggs are additionally key to the Mediterranean Diet, as is fish. Conversely, red meat is eaten just once in a while.

Solid fats

Solid fats are the backbone of the Mediterranean diet. They're eaten rather than fewer sound fats, for example, immersed and trans fats, which add to coronary illness.

Olive oil is the essential wellspring of included fat in the Mediterranean diet. Olive oil gives monounsaturated fat, which has been found to lower total cholesterol and low-thickness lipoprotein (LDL or "awful") cholesterol levels. Nuts and seeds likewise contain monounsaturated fat.

Fish are additionally significant in the Mediterranean eating regimen. Greasy fish —, for example, mackerel, herring, sardines, tuna fish, salmon, and lake trout — are wealthy in omega-3 unsaturated fats, a kind of polyunsaturated fat that may diminish aggravation in the body. Omega-3 unsaturated fats likewise help decline triglycerides, reduce blood coagulating, and decline the danger of stroke and cardiovascular breakdown.

Shouldn't something be said about wine?

The Mediterranean eating regimen ordinarily permits red wine with some restraint. Even though liquor has been related to a diminished danger of coronary illness in specific examinations, it's in no way, shape, or form hazard-free. The Dietary Guidelines for Americans alert against starting to drink or drinking all the more regularly based on potential medical advantages.

Eating the Mediterranean way.

Keen on attempting the Mediterranean diet? These tips will assist you with the beginning:

• Eat more leafy foods. Go for 7 to 10 servings every day of green foods.

• Opt for entire grains. Change to whole grain bread, oat, and pasta. Trial with other entire grains, for example, bulgur and farro.

• Use healthy fats. Attempt olive oil as a trade for spread when cooking. Rather than putting spread or margarine on bread, have a go at dunking it in seasoned olive oil.

• Eat more fish. Eat fish two times every week. Crisp or water-stuffed fish, salmon, trout, mackerel, and herring are sound decisions. Flame-broiled fish tastes great and requires little cleanup. Maintain a strategic distance from southern style fish.

• Reduce red meat: substitute fish, poultry, or beans for beef. If you eat meat, ensure it's lean, and keep parcels little.

• Enjoy some dairy. Eat low-fat Greek or plain yogurt and limited quantities of an assortment of cheeses.

• Spice it up. Herbs and flavors lift season and diminish the requirement for salt.

The Mediterranean eating routine is a good and reliable approach to eat. Numerous individuals who change to this style of eating state they'll never eat some other way.

CHAPTER ONE

WHAT IS MEDITERRANEAN DIET?

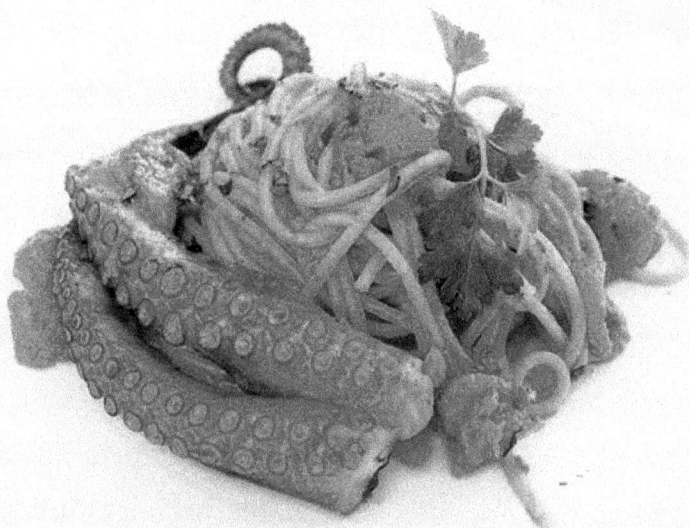

Throughout various ages, onlookers have had the option to perceive that the individuals who populate the district around the Mediterranean Sea live longer lives than do people in some different pieces of the world. Generally, the explanation regularly ascribed to the life span of the individuals of the Mediterranean locale was the atmosphere. In any case, as specialists turned out to be increasingly adroit and as logical strategies turned out to be progressively advanced, it turned out to be evident that while the climate examples of the Mediterranean region, for the most part, were beautiful and welcoming, it was the eating regimen of the individuals in the area that represented their more drawn out lives.

There are various explicit variables identified with the Mediterranean eating routine that nutritionists and therapeutic specialists accept to add to the life span. The more significant of these components are examined inside the limits of this article for your data and direction.

Therapeutic Effects of the Mediterranean Diet

A large number of the particular nourishment things that are a piece of a Mediterranean diet routine are high in enemies of oxidants. Logically, enemies of oxidants are significant mixes found in specific nourishments and refreshments that work to kill the dangerous idea of oxidants or free radicals that are found in the human body. Oxidants or free radicals are delivered when the body consumes oxygen to create vitality. As it were, oxidants indeed can be viewed as waste that dirties the human body.

After some time, the gathering of oxidants in the body quickens the maturing procedure. Cells wear and lose their flexibility. Organs wind up working less productively and successfully. In fact, ongoing logical research has exhibited that oxidants stop up veins raising the risk of stroke. Oxidants are found to add to malignant growth, coronary illness, and diabetes - the significant sicknesses most liable for making individuals have unexpected losses.

The sorts of products of the soil that structure the establishment of the Mediterranean eating regimen - including lavishly hued and verdant green vegetables - which are high in enemies of oxidants, have a remedial and life delaying impact on the average human body.

2. Decreasing Cancer Risks

In many pieces of the world, disease of different sorts is the primary source of sudden passing. Studies embraced by scientists in Europe, Japan, and the United States in the previous thirty years have exhibited that the Mediterranean eating regimen successfully decreases the dangers of specific kinds of malignancies.

An eating regimen that is high in crisp products of the soil has been demonstrated to be successful in decreasing the dangers of a full cluster of various sorts of tumors. As has been noted already, the Mediterranean eating regimen incorporates the liberal utilization of crisp products of the soil.

The Mediterranean eating regimen incorporates almost no creature fat. There is an immediate connection between the utilization of creature fat and colorectal malignancy, perhaps the deadliest type of the infection that customarily ends the lives of individuals in their forties and fifties.

Olive oil (genuinely the establishment of the Mediterranean diet) had been appeared to diminish the danger of bosom malignancy.

By lessening the dangers balanced by malignancy, the life expectancy of people has been appeared to increment apparently in ponders that have pursued gatherings of individuals after some time.

3. Lessening Coronary Heart Disease Risks

Coronary illness is one of the best three reasons for sudden passing all through the world - except in the Mediterranean locale. Specialists have presumed that diet has played a tremendous and significant job in lessening the danger of coronary illness among the individuals who populate the nations encompassing the Mediterranean Sea.

A significant examination in seven nations (Italy, Greece, Yugoslavia, Finland, United States, Netherlands, and Japan) showed that those individuals who pursued a Mediterranean diet routine were less inclined to have coronary illness and were more reluctant to have their lives stopped as a result of genuine and at last lethal heart conditions.

4. Diminishing Hypertension

In some capacity, the jury is still out on the immediate impacts among diet and hypertension or hypertension. It has been exhibited that hypertension and hypertension is liable for unexpected losses the world over. Likewise, there is solid proof to recommend that taking out specific things from an eating routine - like prepared salts - can work to lessen the danger of hypertension.

Furthermore, there is proof to help the suggestion that an eating regimen high in fiber and low in creature fats (like that of the Mediterranean district) attempts to lessen the danger of hypertension and sudden passing from this infection.

5. Diabetes Prevention and Control

The Mediterranean eating routine is appropriate for fighting off the positive impacts of diabetes. The occurrence of sudden passing as a result of diabetes is lower in those locales in which the Mediterranean eating routine is drilled. Since diabetes is an illness that can be controlled through diet, choosing to use the

Mediterranean method can work to add years to an individual's life.

6. The Cumulative Effect of the Mediterranean Diet

Note that the significant impacts of the Mediterranean eating regimen have all the earmarks of being combined after some time. In different words, the more drawn out individual practices the feasting propensities for the Mediterranean arrangement, a higher amount of natural physical advantages of this good dieting routine will be instilled into an individual's cosmetics. The benefits of a Mediterranean eating regimen truly are hidden away after some time, expanding an individual's life expectancy and adding to their general wellbeing and prosperity presently as well into what's to come.

Brief History of the Mediterranean Diet

Lately, a developing number of people in various nations around the globe have gotten progressively worried about their wellbeing. Because of the way that numerous individuals have gained increasingly concerned about their general welfare, these people have given nearer consideration to what they eat all the time. In the last examination, these people are settling on dietary choices intended to improve their general wellbeing and prosperity.

As individuals have gotten progressively aware of their wellbeing and diet, a significant number of these equivalent people have gotten keen on the Mediterranean eating regimen routine. If you are a person who acknowledges the interrelationship among nutrition and wellbeing, you may have a positive enthusiasm for the historical backdrop of the Mediterranean eating routine.

Before you can fittingly comprehend what the Mediterranean eating regimen is about, you have to value that it is, to a greater extent, an idea than a particular feasting schedule. In actuality, there is nothing of the sort as a Mediterranean eating regimen essential to the entirety of the nations in the Mediterranean district of the world. Or maybe, the "Mediterranean eating routine" comprises of those nourishment things that individuals who live in the different countries in the region expend in like manner.

The Origins of the Mediterranean Diet

The idea of the Mediterranean eating routine is gotten from the dietary patterns and examples of the individuals who populate the nations of Italy, Greece, Spain, France, Tunisia, Lebanon, and Morocco. Accordingly, the Mediterranean eating routine incorporates an enormous cluster of tasty nourishment. In the purpose of truth, if an individual chooses to embrace the idea of the Mediterranean feasting plan, or if an individual decides to pursue a Mediterranean eating regimen routine, the person in question will be able to appreciate an exceptional collection of tasty admission.

The eating routine of the people groups that have populated the districts around the Mediterranean Sea has remained about unaltered for well more than one thousand years. The historical backdrop of the area is packed with instances of people living longer than correspondingly arranged individuals who devoured interchange consumes fewer calories. As the centuries progressed, the individuals of the Mediterranean Sea district have delighted in longer lives that individuals in different pieces of the world at the equivalent authentic age.

At the core of the Mediterranean eating regimen are nourishments and drinks that are indigenous to the geographic landmass encompassing the Mediterranean Sea. To put it plainly, the improvement of the Mediterranean slimming down and eating design at first created by fortune. The individuals of the area regularly and justifiably ate those nourishments and drank those drinks that promptly were accessible in their homes.

The Elements of the Mediterranean Diet Scheme

As referenced already, throughout the hundreds of years, the eating routine of the people groups of the Mediterranean Sea locale has remained unaltered. The Mediterranean eating regimen comprises of the abundant utilization of various sound nourishment things including:

* Fresh organic product

* Fresh vegetables

* Low fat nuts

* Whole grains

* Monounsaturated fat

The Mediterranean diet used by individuals for a great many ages prohibits or restrains certain nourishment things that have been regarded as unsafe in ongoing logical thinks about. These not precisely beautiful nourishment things include:

* Saturated fats

* Red and greasy meat

* Rich dairy items

* Oily fish

The Notable Mediterranean Diet Scheme Effects

On the historical backdrop of the Mediterranean eating routine, the individuals who occupy the district have a verifiably lower pace of coronary illness and related sicknesses that, in many cases, have an immediate dietary association. With the appearance of logical examinations that have related the frequency of medical issues with a less than stellar eating routine, the constructive outcomes of the Mediterranean eating routine have become undeniable.

Research throughout the previous two decades has decisively shown that the people who populate the Mediterranean area are burdened with coronary illness and comparative afflictions far less frequently than individuals in different districts of the world. The specialists who have directed these examinations have reasoned that there is a substantial probability that the eating regimen conspire that is normal in the Mediterranean area is answerable for keeping up the great soundness of the individuals who live on that side of the globe all through the previous one thousand years.

During the previous twenty years, a noteworthy number of individuals in various nations around the globe have turned their consideration towards discovering sound eating regimen regimens that are low in saturated fat and that incorporate abundant servings of fresh foods grown from the ground. Subsequently, the Mediterranean eating routine has gotten the attention of multitudinous individuals who need to integrate proper dieting into their general course of sober living. To put it plainly, the Mediterranean eating regimen incorporates nourishments and refreshments that, when devoured with some restraint, can work to decrease the danger of some genuine illnesses and can help in making the critical establishment for a long, healthy lifetime.

Mediterranean Diet Health Benefits

The Mediterranean eating regimen has numerous medical advantages. Pondering specialists have gone through years attempting to find why. Albeit diverse areas have embraced a significantly more westernized eating regimen propensity, which has brought about a mounting heftiness issue, networks that still pursue the customary Mediterranean eating routine keep on encountering wellbeing, which is the jealousy of the western world.

The Mediterranean eating routine comprises principally of crisp, solid plant nourishment like entire grains, vegetables, organic products, nuts, vegetables, olives, fish, and fish. They join this with decreased measures of red meat and dairy items.

The Mediterranean eating regimen is increasingly nutritious because nourishments are less handled. Preparing nourishment, and in any event, cooking, it denies it of supplements. Yet, in a customary Mediterranean eating regimen, most nourishments are eaten crude or gently cooked. At the point when red meat is served, it is generally cut back of abundance excess. The general eating routine gives ample fiber, healthy fats, nutrients, minerals, protein, and essential unsaturated fats required by the body to keep up wellbeing and avert incessant sicknesses like coronary illness and malignancy.

Another essential part of the usual Mediterranean eating routine is that only one out of every odd dinner contains creature tissue (for example, meat or fish). There are regular days with no creature tissue being expended by any means. Nowadays, the protein segment of the supper is gotten from things like beans, nuts, seeds, and eggs. Even though eggs are as yet creature items, late research demonstrates that eggs don't expand blood cholesterol as researchers and specialists used to accept. Another current option in contrast to meat is tofu, which originates from soybeans. While this isn't a piece of the eating regimen, it would positively be a beneficial expansion to it.

These things bring about the Mediterranean eating regimen being high in monounsaturated unsaturated fats, also called M.U.F.As which are solid fats. Diets containing M.U.F.As (and polyunsaturated fats, or P.U.F.As) as opposed to soaked and trans fats, will, in general, give certain medical advantages including the diminished danger of:

• Heart sickness

• High Cholesterol

• Stroke

• Cancer

• Type II Diabetes

• Parkinson's Disease

• Alzheimer's

• Depression

• Metabolic disorder

Let's investigate these.

Decreased danger of coronary illness and elevated Cholesterol

Significant levels of immersed fats bring about expanded cholesterol in the circulatory system. The cholesterol joins to the dividers of veins, causing a narrowing of the supply routes that can prompt blockages, coronary episodes, and coronary illness. The decreased measure of immersed fat in customary Mediterranean eating regimens brings about lower cholesterol levels. Now and again, elevated cholesterol is innate and is brought about by the liver, creating excessively. A solid diet containing high measures of Omega 3 unsaturated fats is demonstrated to battle this issue effectively and can have a considerable bringing down impact on cholesterol levels.

Decreased danger of Stroke

A Columbia University Medical Center study in which scientists pursued 712 members over a multi-year time frame found that members who sought a moderate Mediterranean eating regimen were 21% less inclined to encounter a stroke. Members who pursued a severe eating regimen were 36% more averse to encounter a stroke.

Decreased danger of malignant growth

As indicated by an investigation by the Department of Clinical Sciences, University of Las Palmas de Gran Canaria, Spain: "There is a 'plausible' defensive job of the Mediterranean eating routine toward malignancy when all is said in done." A National Cancer foundation investigation of 500,000 individuals found that individuals who devoured more than 4 oz (113g) of red meat every day were 30% bound to bite the dust from ANY reason more than ten years than the individuals who expended less. Wieners and prepared meats expanded the hazard considerably more.

Reduced Troubles of Diabetes

Use of starches and high fiber nourishments reduces the Glycemic Index of nourishments, and low GI food sources avoid spikes in glucose levels. So a low GI eating routine, for example, the Mediterranean eating routine will in general forestall diabetes... See the area on metabolic disorder beneath

Decreased danger of Parkinson's and Alzheimer's

A few studies demonstrate that individuals who hold fast to the Mediterranean diet have lower paces of Parkinson's and Alzheimer's infections. Scientists are uncertain why this is the situation, yet they accept that sound nourishment decisions improving cholesterol, glucose levels, and vein wellbeing might be the reason.

Diminished danger of Depression

English Researchers contemplated wretchedness and diet over 3,500 moderately aged office laborers for a long while ago. These discoveries showed that people who ate an eating regimen high in handled meat, chocolate, sugar, singed nourishment, refined grains, and high-fat dairy items were bound to endure sadness. Persons who take an eating routine wealthy in organic products, vegetables, and fish like a Mediterranean eating regimen were less inclined to endure sorrow. Their discoveries strengthens other research that has discovered that solid weight control plans can insure against sickness.

Decreased danger of metabolic disorder

Numerous overweight and stout individuals experience the ill effects of a condition called Metabolic Syndrome. A metabolic disorder is a gathering of terms - hypertension, strange glucose levels, exorbitant muscle to fat ratio around the midsection, or irregular cholesterol levels - that happen together. These expand the danger of coronary illness, stroke, and diabetes. People on the Mediterranean eating routine have been seen as less inclined to be overweight along these lines lessening the occurrence of this condition.

Along these lines, as should be obvious, embracing a customary Mediterranean eating regimen has numerous beneficial medical advantages. It has even been found to turn around countless constant ailments, for example, type II diabetes, hypertension, angina, and in any event, improving portability in individuals who experience the ill effects of joint pain. So perhaps it's time you attempted this tasty, sound eating regimen!

The Power of the Mediterranean Diet

The Mediterranean eating routine is the name that has been given to a specific dietary method that was initially utilized by individuals in less affluent areas of Italy and Greece for a long time. This eating routine was not initially thought to be exceptionally sound in these areas, as the individuals ate these nourishments due to need, instead of in light of the Mediterranean eating routine weight reduction and fantastic sustenance benefits they encountered. This sort of food is far not quite the same as what you may anticipate from this district.

However, it is generally a lot more advantageous because things like grease and margarine are seldom utilized.

What It Entails

Essentially, a Mediterranean eating routine calls for individuals to eat a lot of new natural products, plant nourishments, fish, poultry, some dairy items while utilizing additional virgin olive oil as the essential wellspring of fat. Additionally, a reasonable measure of eggs can be eaten every month, while red meat is to be maintained a strategic distance from however much as could reasonably be expected. Red meat can be eaten in low sums, yet suppers ought not to be based on it because of how it influences the heart. The Mediterranean eating routine is intended to bring down the danger of coronary illness since olive oil is high in monounsaturated fats, which have been known to diminish this hazard generously. This additionally decreases the body's cholesterol levels, which is likewise a positive thing for the organization.

History of the Mediterranean Diet

Even though this eating routine was first uncovered in 1945, it didn't generally hit standard levels until the 1990s, when individuals started to build up a newly discovered consciousness of what they were eating. This is around the time that activity shows started showing up on TV, and smart dieting started to become prevalent once more. The Mediterranean eating routine depends on the possibility that individuals in these locales have a much slower pace of coronary illness than individuals with comparative fat admission in different regions of the world. For instance, an individual living in the United States and an individual residing in Greece could spend precisely the same measure of fat quite a long time after a year. Yet, the American would have a higher possibility of experiencing coronary illness since the person is feeling the loss of specific components from their eating routine.

Effects on Health

The principle fixing in a Mediterranean eating routine that is accepted to have the most impact on an individual's wellbeing is additional virgin olive oil. This is because the eating routine is innately low in saturated fat. However, the olive oil makes it high in monounsaturated fat, which (as recently referenced) is useful for your heart. The Mediterranean eating regimen is likewise extremely high in dietary fiber, which advances the normality of the stomach related framework. The eating routine can here, and there be high in salt when it is contained:

• Olives

- Capers

- Salad dressing

- Fish roe

This salt substance isn't a negative thing, notwithstanding, because those things contain common salts, the body can utilize and retain all the more serenely.

Exercise

One thing that numerous individuals probably won't understand about Mediterranean diet weight reduction is that the individuals who begun the eating routine by and large worked outside and reasonably hard. This implies they were getting a lot of activity every single day, notwithstanding outside air. This, in the mix with the little bits these people would eat, prompted slender and solid bodies. This helped heart soundness obviously, which is another motivation behind why they experienced far fewer passings cardiovascular issues.

Restorative Findings

Various medicinal studies have been led on the Mediterranean diet, and they have discovered that men who lived in Crete, which is one of the areas where this eating regimen was initially utilized, had a low frequency of coronary illness. This happened notwithstanding the reality they expended high measures of fats much of the time. One of the principal purposes behind this finding is that a large number of these men changed from margarine to additional virgin olive oil since it was more affordable. They additionally had a high nutrient C admission and decreased the measure of red meat contrasted with different pieces of the globe. It ought to be noticed that the discoveries of this examination were sensational to the point that the outcomes were distributed before the investigation had been finished. This was because the individuals who were leading the test didn't accept they could hush up about the data anymore. Different sicknesses and ailments which have been entirely influenced by this eating routine incorporate osteoporosis, limiting the danger of certain types of malignancy, hypersensitivities, Alzheimer's illness, and more studies are being attempted as I compose this article.

Weight reduction

Further studies have demonstrated occasions of Mediterranean diet weight reduction, as 322 individuals took an interest in an investigation where a few people were dependent upon a low-carb diet, others embraced a low-fat diet, and some ate just a Mediterranean diet. The outcomes indicated that the individuals who were on the Mediterranean eating regimen had the best weight reduction of all, with the main two members losing 12 and 10 pounds separately. The investigation featured that Mediterranean eating regimen weight reduction is viable and ought to be considered by any individual who is experiencing difficulty getting in shape.

Why Choose the Mediterranean Lifestyle

The Mediterranean eating routine isn't only an approach to shed pounds, yet it is an approach to altogether wholly change you, and in doing as such, dragging out it. The medical advantages are constant, particularly when they are joined with work out, making this sustenance experience something undoubtedly worth investigating. The primary concern is - the individuals who are on this eating regimen have lower death rates than the individuals who are not, which is reason enough to try it out. If that you have a background marked by coronary illness in your family, you indeed can't bear to proceed similarly, and now you have another option.

Mediterranean Diet Food Pyramid Vs Traditional Food Pyramid

For a large portion of us, the most perceived image of sound nourishment is found in the nourishment pyramid. It demonstrates which nourishments we ought to eat in which part measures with the goal that our body gets the supplements it requires. In case you're making a sound eating regimen plan, you would do well to take a gander at the Mediterranean eating routine nourishment pyramid. The Mediterranean eating routine is perceived as perhaps the most advantageous eating regimen on the planet and is supported by the Mayo Clinic.

What is the Mediterranean Diet Food Pyramid?

The Mediterranean eating routine nourishment pyramid is an option in contrast to the conventional one, which is turning out to be progressively famous because it did not depend on prominent nourishment patterns. The eating routine itself is established on a great many long periods of convention inside the Mediterranean area. The dietary assemblies of Mediterranean nations have, for some time, been perceived as exceptionally sound, and the nourishment that they devour is one of the primary factors in that strength. Knowing the contrast between the conventional nourishment pyramid and the Mediterranean one will help you in improving your wellbeing.

The Mediterranean eating regimen nourishment pyramid is necessarily unique to the conventional one with which we are recognizable. There are sure glaring contrasts, to be specific;

• The Mediterranean one doesn't have a fats classification.

• Red meat is at the highest point of the Mediterranean pyramid as nourishment to eat least of alongside desserts/pastries.

• Olive oil is assembled with the foods grown from the ground as something to be devoured now and again.

The top part of the Mediterranean eating routine nourishment pyramid begins with red meat as a wellspring of creature protein. Red meat and desserts are the least devoured nourishments in the Mediterranean, around 2-3 times each month. The following classification, expended two or three times each week, is poultry, eggs, and dairy items like cheddar and yogurt. Next, fish are consumed practically day by day. Essentially, the Mediterranean eating routine is low in immersed fats and high in monounsaturated fats and omega 3.

The base degree of the pyramid is made out of natural products, vegetables, vegetables (beans), nuts, seeds, herbs, flavors, whole grain bread, entire grain pasta, couscous, dark colored rice, polenta, and other entire grains. Individuals in the Mediterranean once in a while eat handled grains (for example, white flour). An enormous assortment of these new nourishments are consumed every day, and they are generally either crude or delicately cooked. This implies the supplements are as yet unblemished. Preparing nourishments slaughters most supplements or renders them indigestible. Thus it is in every case better to eat nourishment crude or incompletely cooked.

The last piece of the Mediterranean pyramid is the proposal of six glasses of water for every day and a reasonable measure of wine (for example, one glass of red wine with supper).

It is fascinating to take note of that olive oil is gathered with the products of the soil in the Mediterranean pyramid. As you can envision, olive oil is an enormous piece of the Mediterranean eating routine, and numerous dishes contain it. While the facts demonstrate that oil is high in calories, olive oil is a healthy monounsaturated fat that is high in cancer prevention agents and contains omega three, so we can devour somewhat more as long as we don't go over the edge. Monounsaturated oils like olive oil are mitigating and are useful for illnesses like asthma and joint inflammation. They're likewise heart-solid because the omega 3 brings down LDL ("terrible") cholesterol, and raises HDL ("great") cholesterol. The soundest olive oil is additional virgin olive oil.

You might be thinking about how individuals in the Mediterranean get their iron since they don't eat a great deal of red meat. The response to this is equivalent to it would be for a veggie lover. Vegetables (beans) and verdant green vegetables are likewise great wellsprings of iron, and the Mediterranean eating routine is loaded with these solid nourishments. The entire Mediterranean eating routine nourishment pyramid comprises sound nourishments guaranteeing that the individuals who pursue the Mediterranean eating routine experience ideal wellbeing.

Five Reasons Why the Mediterranean Diet is a Healthy Choice

If that you are someone who has been on the chase for a healthy eating regimen plan, you may feel overpowered a significant part of the time. In the 21st century, it is about outlandish for an individual to turn on a TV or open a paper without being assaulted with promotions for a wide range of diet plans and items.

With the large cluster of diet plans, projects, enhancements, and helps available, it can appear to be about awkward to choose an eating regimen plan that can and will best address your issues now and into what's to come. All the more critically, it very well may be difficult to recognize if that some of these different eating routine plots is a sound course to seek after. In numerous cases, prevailing fashion counts calories indeed are not founded based on stable living.

As you go ahead thinking about what sort of diet plan or routine will best serve your inclinations and improve your wellbeing into the future, you will need to investigate the advantages that can be had through the Mediterranean eating regimen.

While there are various reasons why the Mediterranean eating regimen is a sound methodology, there are five essential reasons why the Mediterranean eating routine is a decent decision.

1. The Benefits of Fruits, Vegetable, Fiber, and Whole Grains

A significant segment of the Mediterranean diet incorporates the customary utilization of crisp products of the soil. Restorative specialists and nutritionists generally concur that an individual ought to eat somewhere in the range of five and six servings of new products of the soil (or steamed things) every day.

Individuals who hold fast to the Mediterranean eating regimen wind up eating more than the base prescribed stipend of leafy foods. Accordingly, nutritionists in various pieces of the world have taken to prescribing a Mediterranean based eating routine to their customers. Also, specialists who counsel with their patients about smart dieting rehearses generally end up prescribing the Mediterranean eating regimen these days.

Past foods are grown from the ground, and the Mediterranean diet incorporates sound measures of dietary fiber and entire grains. Fiber and whole grains have demonstrated influential in bringing down the occurrence of coronary illness and a few sorts of malignancy.

2. The Benefits of Olive Oil - Avoiding Saturated Fat

A few people have a fundamental misperception about the Mediterranean diet. These people have heard that the Mediterranean eating regimen is high in fat. In some capacity, there is a trace of validity in the origination that the Mediterranean eating routine is more top in fat than are some other eating fewer carbs programs. An individual after the Mediterranean diet takes in around 30% of their daily calories from fat. (Most foods suggested the admission of calories from fat at the pace of about thirteen to fifteen percent for each day. Nonetheless, these weight control plans are examining the ingesting of creature fat.)

By far, most of the fat that an individual on the Mediterranean eating routine devours originates from olive oil. As it were, the fat found in the Mediterranean eating regimen isn't the risky immersed fat that can cause sickness, obesity, and other wellbeing concerns. Inquire about has exhibited that there are various substantial advantages to devouring olive oil, including a decrease in the danger of the rate of bosom malignant growth in ladies.

3. Dairy in Moderation

While the usage of low or non-fat dairy stuffs with some restraint can be valuable in certain occurrences, numerous individuals the world over depend on overwhelming creams, eggs, and other fat-filled dairy items in their everyday consumes fewer calories. The Mediterranean eating routine is low in dairy. For sure, any dairy items that are incorporated inside the eating routine is low fat. An individual is viewed as an amazingly substantial egg consumer if that the person in question devours four eggs in seven days.

4. Red Meat in Moderation

There are almost no red meat is included inside the Mediterranean eating regimen. With regards to meat things, this eating routine depends on reasonable measures of lean poultry and crisp fish. Accordingly, individuals who pursue the

Mediterranean eating regimen plan have lower levels of "awful" cholesterol and more elevated levels of "good: cholesterol.

What's more, as a result of the incorporation of lean, crisp fish in the eating routine, disciples to the Mediterranean eating routine appreciate the counter oxidant benefits that are found in certain fish oils and items.

5. A Well Balanced Dieting Scheme

In the last examination, the Mediterranean eating regimen is picking up praise from specialists and disciples the world over because it is a good consuming fewer calories program. Many studies exhibit that a decent diet that is low in fat and that incorporates organic products, vegetables, entire grains, and lean meat attempts to guarantee all out wellbeing and health.

The Mediterranean Diet isn't an eating routine, fundamentally yet a free term alluding to the dietary facts of the individuals in the Mediterranean district. Every nation that outskirts the Mediterranean Sea offers a variation to the Mediterranean Diet. Contrasts in the ethnic foundation, culture, horticultural generation, and religion between the Mediterranean nations make the variety in every nation's eating routine. In any case, each diet offers various qualities that are normal to the entirety of the Mediterranean countries.

The Mediterranean Diet has high utilization of organic products, vegetables, beans, nuts, seeds, bread, and different grains. Generally, products of the soil are privately developed in the Mediterranean Diet. Products of the earth frequently are devoured crude or negligibly prepared. Foods grown from the ground contain numerous essential nutrients and minerals just as cancer prevention agents that are critical for good wellbeing.

The Mediterranean Diet's essential wellspring of fat is as monounsaturated fat. Olive oil is a monounsaturated fat that is a rich wellspring of cancer prevention agents, including nutrient E. Olive oil is utilized rather than spread, margarine, and different fats. Indeed, range and cream are used just on uncommon events. Olive oil in the Mediterranean Diet is utilized to get ready tomato sauces, vegetable dishes, servings of mixed greens, and to broil fish.

The Mediterranean Diet energizes reduced admission of fish; however, practically no entry of meat. Red meat and poultry are expended just sparingly. Fish is the meat of decision. Around 5-15 oz. of slick fish, individually, are consumed week after week. Slick fish incorporates fish, mackerel, salmon, trout, herring, and sardines. Sleek fish are an incredible wellspring of omega-3 unsaturated fats.

Dairy items are devoured in low to direct sums. Dairy items from an assortment of creatures, for example, goats, sheep, bison, bovines, and camels, are fundamentally devoured as low-fat cheddar and yogurt. Next to no fresh milk is eaten. Dinners are typically joined by wine or water.

The Mediterranean Diet urges low to direct utilization of wine. Wine is typically overcome with a dinner. The sort of wine devoured is usually red wine, which contains a rich wellspring of phytonutrients. Among the phytonutrients, polyphenols, mainly, are significant cell reinforcements. Studies have shown that people who have a light to direct utilization of liquor live longer than nondrinkers. One mixed drink (1.5 oz. refined spirits, 5 oz. wine, 12 oz. lager) every day for ladies and two blended beverages day by day for men is viewed as moderate admission of liquor.

If that you wish to join the Mediterranean Diet into your life, here are a couple of recommendations. Foods grown from the ground ought to be of a wide assortment. You should go after at any rate 7-10 servings of entire products of the soil day by day. You ought to dodge any vegetables that are set up in margarine or cream sauces. High fiber bread, grains, and pasta are expended every day. This incorporates dark colored rice, wheat, whole grain bread, and oat. You ought to evade desserts, white bread, scones, breadsticks, and any refined starches.

Protein admission is low in immersed fat. Protein admission from red meat is of lean cuts, poultry without the skin, and low-fat dairy nourishments (skim milk, yogurt). You ought to dodge bacon, sausage, and other prepared or high-fat meat. You should also like to maintain a strategic distance from milk or cheddar that isn't low fat.

The admission of fish is 1-2 times week after week from sleek fish, flaxseed, pecans, and spinach. Stable oils (additional virgin olive oil, canola oil, flaxseed oil) are utilized for cooking, serving of mixed greens dressings, and different employments. You ought to stay away from omega-6 fats, for example, corn, sunflower, safflower, soybean, and shelled nut. You're eating regimen ought to likewise incorporate peas, beans, soy, lentils, tree nuts (almonds, walnuts, pecans, Brazil nuts), and vegetables. You ought to stay away from vigorously salted or nectar broiled nuts.

A moderate admission of liquor with the night supper is discretionary. The Mediterranean Diet accentuates entire regular nourishments. This implies staying away from cheap food, singed nourishment, margarine, chips, saltines, prepared merchandise, doughnuts, or any handled nourishments that contain Trans unsaturated fats.

The Mediterranean style diets are near the dietary rules of the American Heart Association. Diets of the Mediterranean individuals contain a moderately high level of fat calories, about 40%. The American Heart Association embraces an eating routine that includes about 30% fat admission. Be that as it may, the healthy Mediterranean Diet has less immersed fat than the typical American eating routine.

Analysts are presently attempting to conclude the parts of the Mediterranean Diet that are liable for the Mediterranean populaces' more extended future contrasted with other European populaces. Be that as it may, the consolidated impacts of various fixings, for example, a casual eating disposition, a lot of daylight, and progressively physical movement, are probably going to contribute to the general robust way of life of the Mediterranean area. The Mediterranean Diet has a lower occurrence of coronary illness and disease, which makes the Mediterranean Diet a public decent decision in wellbeing.

CHAPTER TWO

HISTORY OF MEDITERRANEAN DIET

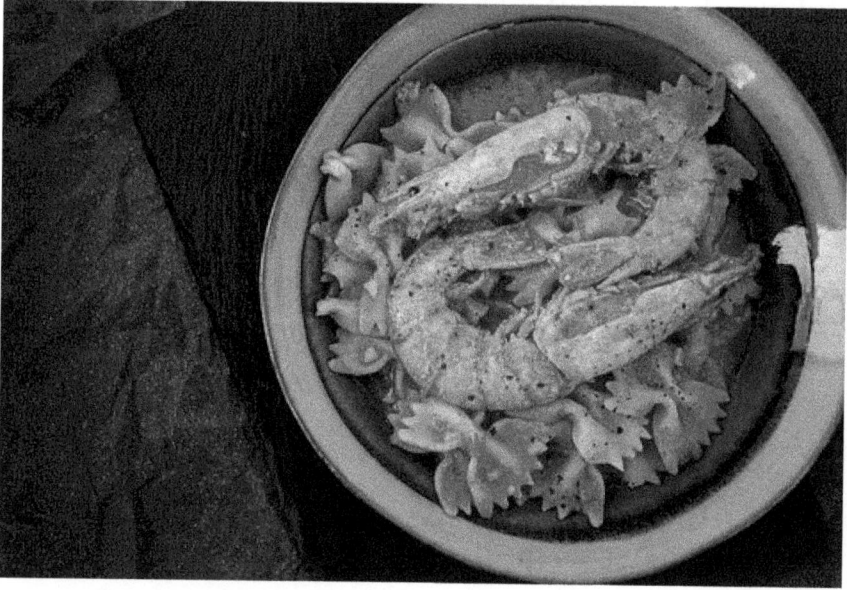

The Mediterranean convention offers a cuisine wealthy in hues, smells, and recollections, which bolster the taste and the soul of the individuals who live in agreement with nature. Everybody is discussing the Mediterranean eating regimen, yet few are the individuals who do it appropriately, in this way producing a great deal of perplexity in the peruse. Thus for some, it corresponds with the pizza, others distinguished it with the noodles with meat sauce, in a blend of pseudo recorded customs and legends that don't comprehend the inquiry that is at the premise of any eating regimen: join, and parity the nourishment to fulfill the subjective and quantitative needs of an individual and one might say, protects his wellbeing using substances that help the body to perform ordinary crucial capacities. The motivation behind our work is to show that the blend of taste and wellbeing is an objective that can be done by everyone, regardless of the individuals who accept that lone a liberal caloric admission can ensure the integrity of a dish and the fulfillment of the purchasers. That ought not to be an outright curiosity, since the sound customs of the Mediterranean cooking, we have utilized for quite a while in a wide assortment of delectable gastronomic decisions, from welcoming hues and solid fragrances and following wellbeing.

Time appears to stop on the island of Pantelleria, situated on the Mediterranean Sea, around 36 miles from North Africa and 65 miles from the bank of Sicily. There are no taxicabs that advance around the border of this little island—just 9 miles in length and 6 miles wide—made out of coal-black volcanic rocks, leftovers of old volcanoes, compared against the ocean's green waters. A great many worn dark shake porches wind around slants, looking like numerous levels on a wedding cake. Conventional low stone bungalows, formed in colored stone and vaulted white arches, called "dammuso," speck the slopes. Local people—just 8,000 of them—are warm and lively, having the moderate and loosened up nature so pervasive in this piece of the world.

Barely any vacationers have found this "dark pearl" in the Mediterranean, even though it's become a mystery hideaway for planners and engineers, including Giorgio Armani, who built up a manor there. One of Pantelleria's most enchanting properties in the neighborhood cooking, which spotlights on territorially created plant nourishments, for example, olives, escapades, and herbs and flavors, beholding back to social nourishment customs went down through the ages—the establishment of the Mediterranean diet.

Pantelleria fills in as a clear case of the sorts of nourishments to eat when following the Mediterranean eating regimen. Dinners are made with olive oil, grains, and fresh foods grown from the ground, beans, vegetables, fish, and shellfish. Peruse on to find out about this modern nation's rich history, how the Mediterranean eating routinely advanced, and how following such an eating style can promote ideal wellbeing and prosperity.

Molding the Land for Survival

The conventional eating regimen in the nations encompassing the Mediterranean Sea, including France, Italy, Spain, Morocco, and Greece, was viewed as a "poor man's" diet, created throughout the hundreds of years as individuals worked to make sustenance is less accommodating landscape. In Pantelleria, occupants during ancient occasions chased and raised animals, yet beginning in the Bronze Age, and they bit by bit cleared the island for cultivating, which has been the occupants' essential wellspring of sustenance from the beginning of time and even up to today.

A thousand years back, local people started heaping magma stones to shape miles of impeccably developed dividers that bend around the island. Every incline of each slope was terraced in a bright endeavor to contain and shield the dirt from disintegration, and catch each drop of valuable dampness on this desert island. The porches made a one of a kind biological system, where low grapevines and escapade plants prosper in their brutal environment, as indicated by Gabriella Giuntoli, an honor winning modeler, urban organizer, and master of Pantelleria engineering, who talked at the Old ways International Mediterranean Symposium on September 9, 2012, in Pantelleria. Today, the porches fill in as an effortless, enchanting element of Pantelleria vistas just as a commonsense apparatus for cultivating.

"There was minimal arable land—the island has restricted seaside planes flanked by enormous mountains, and the atmosphere is extraordinary with sporadic precipitation. The breezes blow constantly," said Mary Taylor Simeti, a Sicilian nourishment master who has composed broadly on nourishment customs of the area, and who talked at the meeting.

Another farming and design highlight emerged on the island: the Giardino pantesco, a dry stone walled in area, either round, square, or oval molded, which made the perfect interior climactic conditions required for developing citrus, a natural product. Going back to the Arab mastery of the island, more than 1,500 of these delightful, encased "mystery" plants still exist in Pantelleria.

While these building fortunes draw in gratefulness for their rural appeal, their genuine worth is the showcase of man's mission for endurance by molding the land and condition to continue the body and soul. This aspect is found in the nations along the Mediterranean. In Pantelleria, for instance, the individuals needed to confront a rough territory, low precipitation, and consistent breezes that shook the island. So the patios and encased nurseries made support against the breeze while at the same time enabling dampness from the dew to gather on the stones to give hydration to the dried plants, with no type of water system. These patios and encased nurseries are symbols symbolizing the resourcefulness and assurance that was expected to make the provincial eating regimens in the Mediterranean.

Plants of Pantelleria

Behind the patios, the plants, from olive trees to grapevines, develop low to the ground on a level plane, shielded from the breeze. At the base of every vine, you'll locate a little bowl, which gathers the dew that slides down into the underlying foundations of the grapevine—a procedure that was built many years back.

Pantelleria is acclaimed for Passito di Pantelleria, an old sweet wine going back 2,000 years. It's produced using the Muscat of Alexandria grape (called Zibibbo in Pantelleria), which began from the Nile Delta. This carefully sweet wine is produced using crisp grape must and raisins; wooden racks of grapes drying in the sun can be discovered everywhere throughout the island at gather time.

Other nearby fortunes incorporate tricks, which grow like weeds in the most remote spots, similar to a break in a stone hanging over the ocean. Pantellerians are very glad for their tricks, which are known to be particularly exceptional in taste, "with kinds of the center of the ocean," as indicated by nearby escapade cultivators. The jokes are the bloom buds, which rise out of long trailing vines with coin-formed leaves, gathered by hand before they open into white-purple blooms. Dissimilar to most tricks found in America, Pantellerian escapades are aged and saved in ocean salt rather than vinegar.

This wouldn't be a Mediterranean nation without the nearness of the olive tree, an image of the vegetable world joining the three religions in this area: Christianity, Judaism, and Islam. Yet, in Pantelleria, olive trees appear as little hedges close to 2 ft tall, becoming out as opposed to up.

"If individuals didn't develop it in Pantelleria, they didn't eat it. This is valid for most of the nourishments in the Mediterranean eating routine. The unforgiving atmosphere constrains the yields that can be delivered. However, it's liable for giving them exceptional flavors. There were mind-blowing imagination and imaginativeness in the eating routine here," Simeti stated, posting tomatoes, zucchinis, peppers, potatoes, and wild herbs as regular vegetables developed on the island alongside staples, for example, wheat, grain, lentils, and chickpeas, which went to the Sicilian area in the Neolithic Age. Almonds, which appear in numerous provincial dishes, generally are developed in one's home nursery.

The Birth of Local Dishes

In the same way as other nations in the Mediterranean, the nearby diet in Pantelleria has been molded by a rich history of different ethnic societies, from Arabian to Italian. The locale consistently has been a junction for some human advancements and organizations. While the island was made by volcanic emissions somewhere in the range of 250,000 years prior, the primary pioneers landed from North Africa in 3,000 BC. The Phoenicians and the Carthaginians visited the island, and the Romans involved it in the third century BC.

For quite a long time, privateers looted the island. However, Muslim ranchers colonized it in 860 AD and presented grapes and citrus trees. In 1090, the Arabs were banished, and the island changed hands various occasions throughout the following a very long time until it, at last, was known as Pantelleria. During the Napoleonic wars, French cooking was brought to the Sicilian area, which was hitched with the nearby nourishment custom.

Customary dishes reflected the immense social impacts and nourishment accessibility. Take, for instance, a Pantellerian fish couscous, which owes vigorously to the flavors and customs of North Africa. "A dish with tomatoes, eggplant, and potatoes is an ideal impression of the cooking style of the island. You previously took a gander at your nursery, and afterward, you chose what your formula would be," Simeti said. "While fish is a significant piece of the eating routine here, Pantellerians are a greater number of ranchers than the angler. The dishes were made of straightforward fixings, as it was costly to import nourishments. For instance, sugar was costly to import, such a significant number of the conventional treats were seasoned with nectar or grape must."

During a visit to Pantelleria, you're probably going to see a few notable dishes, including a pesto made of crude tomatoes, olive oil, garlic, and basil; fish couscous with an assortment of nearby fish, vegetables, and vegetables; caponata designed with eggplant, escapades, and olive oil; ciaku ciuka, a mix of eggplant, tomatoes, and potatoes; and Pantescan serving of mixed greens made with potatoes, tomatoes, red onions, and tricks. These neighborhood nourishments are healthy, natural, and liberally seasoned with methods, olive oil, and wild herbs—essential harvests of the island.

The ascent of the Mediterranean Diet for Health

Wellbeing specialists and sustenance scientists didn't make the Mediterranean eating regimen in a lab. "The Mediterranean eating regimen is a customary eating regimen that developed more than 5,000 years," said Antonia Trichopoulou, MD, Ph.D., a teacher at the University of Athens and one of the leading Mediterranean eating regimen analysts who went to the gathering. "Individuals utilized neighborhood assets and arranged nourishment from nothing to create it. It was formed by provincial conditions, culture, and strict practices. Individuals consistently accepted the Mediterranean eating regimen was beneficial for you, yet it hadn't been recorded previously. It's a method for a living—it regards the earth and religions. The emphasis is on occasional nourishments, customary choices, and neighborhood items."

The Mediterranean eating regimen has been the subject of concentrated research for over 50 years, as far back as Ancel Keys, Ph.D., a teacher from the University of Minnesota, first played out his incredible, post-World War II Seven Countries Study, which inspected the wellbeing results of about 13,000 moderately aged men in the United States, Japan, Italy, Greece, the Netherlands, Finland, and afterward Yugoslavia. His group found that men from Crete experienced lower cardiovascular illness rates than their partners in different nations—a connection the specialists credited to the men's after war "poor" diet, which concentrated on natural products, vegetables, grains, beans, and fish.

Since Keys' first perception decades back, many examinations have recorded a variety of medical advantages connected with the conventional Mediterranean eating regimen, including expanded life expectancy; stable weight; improved mind work; less manifestations of rheumatoid joint inflammation and reduced richness and eye wellbeing; lower dangers of specific malignancies, coronary illness, Alzheimer's ailment, and diabetes; and lower levels of circulatory strain and LDL cholesterol.

"The Lyon Diet Heart Trial in 1998 demonstrated that following three years on the Mediterranean eating routine subjects had a 56% lower danger of biting the dust and a half to 70% decreased danger of dead myocardial tissue," said Kathy McManus, MS, RD, LDN, chief of the sustenance division at Brigham and Women's Hospital in Boston, as she featured a portion of the significant clinical discoveries at the symposium.1,2 "In the Gissi Prevenzione Trial in Italy, with more than 11,000 people, the eating regimen was related to a half-diminished demise rate. Presently the eating regimen is the therapeutic standard for weight reduction in diabetes," she said.1, 2

Research on the medical advantages of the Mediterranean eating routine keeps on developing, with the ongoing production of an examination that pulled in overall consideration. In the milestone multicenter PREDIMED preliminary, scientists from Spain found that a Mediterranean eating routine that included nuts diminished the danger of cardiovascular sickness by 30% and explicitly diminished the threat of stroke by 49% when contrasted and a low-fat American Heart Association-suggested diet.3

The exercise of the Mediterranean eating regimen is that it is anything but an enchantment slug—it's not around one specific nourishment that offers extraordinary advantages. It's tied in with eating a basic, plant-based eating regimen, in light of local, nearby, supplement thick nourishments. It's tied in with enjoying the kinds of nourishments and capitalizing on the nourishments accessible to us. These are exercises that can be applied to eats less the nation over. You can eat a neighborhood, regular, plant-rich eating regimen in the Northwest just as in the South, and give uncommon consideration to local dishes, for example, wild mushroom risotto and crisp berry compote in the Northwest and greens with dark looked at peas in the South. By interpreting the critical qualities of the Mediterranean eating routine into our customers' ways of life, we can carry the advantages of this way of life to America.

What's to think about the Mediterranean eating routine?

The Mediterranean eating regimen depends principally on the dietary patterns of southern European nations, with an accentuation on plant nourishments, olive oil, fish, poultry, beans, and grains. There is no single Mediterranean eating regimen; however, the idea draws together the standard nourishment types and empowering propensities from the conventions of various districts, including Crete, Greece, Spain, southern France, Portugal, and Italy.

More research is expected to affirm the exact advantages of the eating regimen. Yet, it is known to be low in trans fats, and free from refined oils and exceptionally prepared meats and nourishments.

These things have been connected to conditions, for example, obesity, diabetes, malignant growth, and cardiovascular infection.

Quick realities about the Mediterranean diet

• There is nobody Mediterranean eating routine. It comprises nourishments from various nations and locales, including Spain, Greece, and Italy.

• The Mediterranean eating regimen is an incredible method to supplant the saturated fats in the typical American eating regimen.

• There is an accentuation on organic products, vegetables, lean meats, and conventional sources.

• It is connected to excellent heart wellbeing, security against maladies, for example, stroke, and avoidance of diabetes.

• Moderation is as yet advised, as the eating routine has a high-fat substance.

• The Mediterranean eating routine ought to be combined with a functioning way of life for the best outcomes.

Diet

The Mediterranean eating routine is an approach to guarantee nourishment originates from a scope of natural, restorative sources.

The Mediterranean eating regimen comprises of:

• High amounts of vegetables, for example, tomatoes, kale, broccoli, spinach, carrots, cucumbers, and onions

• Fresh, natural product, for example, apples, bananas, figs, dates, grapes, and melons.

• High utilization of vegetables, beans, nuts, and seeds, for example, almonds, pecans, sunflower seeds, and cashews

• Whole grains, for example, entire wheat, oats, grain, buckwheat, corn, and dark-colored rice

• Olive oil as the primary wellspring of dietary fat, close by olives, avocados, and avocado oil

• Cheese and yogurt as the primary dairy nourishments, including Greek yogurt

• Moderate measures of fish and poultry, for example, chicken, duck, turkey, salmon, sardines, and clams

• Eggs, including chicken, quail, and duck eggs

• Limited sums of red meats and desserts

• Around one glass for each day of wine, with water as the principle refreshment of decision and no carbonated and improved beverages

This emphasis on plant nourishments and standard sources implies that the Mediterranean eating routine contains supplements, for example,

Energizing fats: The Mediterranean diet is known to be low in immersed fat and high in monounsaturated fat. Dietary rules for the United States prescribe that saturated fat should make up close to 10 percent of calorie admission.

Fiber: The eating regimen is high in fiber, which advances substantial assimilation and is accepted to lessen the danger of inside malignant growth and cardiovascular infection.

High nutrient and mineral substance: Fruits and vegetables give essential nutrients and minerals, which control substantial forms. What's more, the nearness of lean meats gives nutrients, for example, B-12 that are not found in plant nourishments.

Low sugar: The eating regimen is high in common as opposed to include sugar, for instance, in new natural products. Added sugar expands calories without nourishing advantage, is connected to diabetes and hypertension, and happens in a significant number of the handled nourishments missing from the Mediterranean diet.

It is hard to give accurate dietary data on the Mediterranean eating routine since there is no single Mediterranean eating regimen. This is because an assortment of societies and locales is included.

The source and history of the Mediterranean eating regimen

The name of the famous and sound Mediterranean eating regimen, Med Diet, originates from two words that we will dissect, so we will all have a superior connection and comprehension of the eating routine we embraced and will pursue.

Mediterranean: is the name of the ocean that is between Europe, Asia, and Africa, with one regular section from the Atlantic Ocean on the West and an artificial exit on the East towards the Red Sea. The name of the ocean verifiably goes to the Latin's, as in the center of the third century Solinos, was the first to name the sea - Mare Mediterraneum, meaning the sea in the middle of two mainlands and in this way turning into the support or the supporter of the name. (Note that "Mare" implies the ocean in Latin).

It is in the nations encompassing the Mediterranean that we see the foundation of the Mediterranean eating routine. It is in this locale that the Olive trees developed in wealth, organic products were in season during the four seasons because of the mellow atmosphere, and fish was a piece of the eating routine and angling an occupation by most. Furthermore, the Mediterranean herbs were utilized for cooking as well as were being used for Medicinal purposes also in this manner, sparing people groups' lives.

It was additionally in the Mediterranean Sea that the majority of the old civic establishments prospered and from the Mediterranean Sea that incredible Empires like the Roman Empire have begun.

Diet: Our connection and responsibility to the Mediterranean eating routine can turn out to be much more grounded if that we explain the importance of the word " diet". Regularly the word " diet" bears something negative it and it is related to constrained nourishment, coming about because of a neurotic express that one gets into or from the excessive increment of fat or undesired mass in the body. This anyway isn't the situation for the Mediterranean eating routine in such a case that we take a gander at the root of the word " diet" we find that it begins from the Greek word "diaita" which means lifestyle, a method for living.

So the old Greek word for "diet", Diaita, implied " method for living" when all is said in done and was neither alluding nor confined to the dietary needs and propensities for individuals. Instead, it had to do with the entire range of our life: work, rest, buddies, social condition, exercises, and a spot of living.

"Diaita" in antiquated Greece implied the method for living. Along these lines of life was managed off-kilter for the Greeks by God Dias, Zeus, accordingly, the word has its underlying foundations, since he, Dias, was the person who directed and made the conditions from which home, work, nourishment, rest and dress were administered.

So when we pursue the Mediterranean eating routine, we acknowledge to seek a sound method for living that would redundant outcome to lost weight, but instead, it would manage a technique for living that will place us in the right way/track of a long haul reliable result.

The Mediterranean eating routine exists for a long time, and one can contend that it is the most seasoned eating routine on the planet, having an existence of more than 3,000 years. Anyway, the Mediterranean eating routine and method for living for the Western world and explicitly for the US individuals was rediscovered by and is credited to the nutritionist Ancel Keys. This was a thrilling disclosure that has driven American researchers to set up in the late 60s and across the board program of preventive medication on the examinations led by Keys, in this way we have the birth and spread of the Mediterranean Diet.

The Mediterranean eating regimen depends on the conventional nourishments that individuals used to eat in nations like Italy and Greece in 1960.

Scientists noticed that these individuals were outstandingly stable contrasted with Americans and had a generally safe of numerous ways of life sicknesses.

Various studies have now demonstrated that the Mediterranean diet can cause weight reduction and help forestall coronary failures, strokes, type 2 diabetes, and unexpected passing.

There is nobody right approach to pursue the Mediterranean eating regimen, as there are numerous nations around the Mediterranean ocean, and individuals in various zones may have eaten different nourishments. This usually portrays the dietary example usually recommended in contemplates that propose it's a sound method for eating.

CHAPTER THREE

BENEFITS OF MEDITERRANEAN DIET

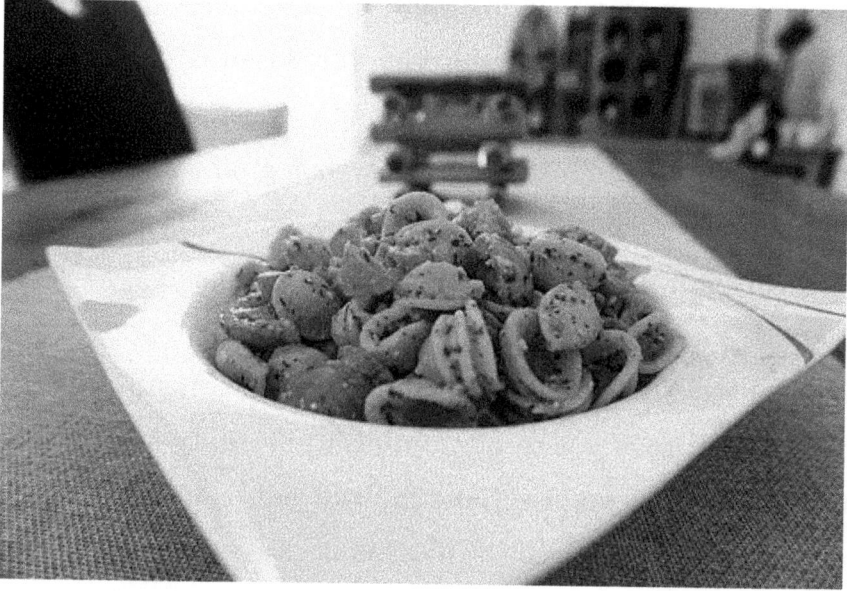

When we are considering Mediterranean nourishment, your psyche may go-to pizza and pasta from Italy or sheep cleaves from Greece. Yet, these dishes don't fit into the solid dietary plans publicized as "Mediterranean." A genuine Mediterranean eating regimen depends on the locale's customary natural products, vegetables, beans, nuts, fish, olive oil, and dairy—with maybe a glass or two of red wine. That is how the occupants of Crete, Greece, and southern Italy ate around 1960, when their paces of interminable malady were among the most reduced on the planet and their future among the most elevated, notwithstanding having just constrained restorative administrations.

What's more, the genuine Mediterranean eating routine is about something other than eating new, healthy meals. Everyday actions and imparting suppers to others are essential components of the Mediterranean Diet Pyramid. Together, they can profoundly affect your mindset and psychological well-being and assist you with encouraging profound gratefulness for the delights of eating well and scrumptious nourishments.

Making changes to your eating regimen is infrequently simple, particularly in case you're attempting to move away from the accommodation of prepared and takeout nourishments. In any case, the Mediterranean eating routine can be economical just as a refreshing and reliable approach to eating. Switching from pepperoni and pasta, and to fish, and avocados may require some exertion. However, you could before long be on the way to a more advantageous and longer life.

Medical advantages of a Mediterranean diet

A conventional Mediterranean eating regimen comprising of enormous amounts of new foods grown from the ground, nuts, fish and olive oil—combined with physical movement—can lessen your danger of genuine mental and physical medical issues by:

Anticipating coronary illness and strokes. Following a Mediterranean diet restrains your admission of refined bread, prepared nourishments, and red meat, and energizes drinking red wine rather than hard alcohol—all factors that can help counteract coronary illness and stroke.

Keeping you deft. In case you're a more grown-up, the supplements chosen with a Mediterranean eating routine may decrease your danger of creating muscle shortcoming and different indications of delicacy by around 70 percent.

Lessening the danger of Alzheimer's. The research proposes that the Mediterranean eating regimen may improve cholesterol, glucose levels, and generally speaking vein wellbeing, which like this, may decrease your danger of Alzheimer's ailment or dementia.

Splitting the danger of Parkinson's sickness. The high levels of cancer prevention agents in the Mediterranean eating regimen can keep cells from experiencing a harming procedure called oxidative pressure, in this way, cutting the danger of Parkinson's infection down the middle.

Increasing life span. By reducing your danger of possessing coronary illness or malignancy with the Mediterranean eating routine, you're lessening your risk of death at any age by 20%.

Ensuring against type 2 diabetes. A Mediterranean diet is wealthy in fiber, which processes gradually, averts large swings in glucose, and can assist you with keeping up a healthy weight.

Significant Benefits of the Mediterranean Diet

The Mediterranean eating regimen revolved around organic products, vegetables, olive oil, nuts, vegetables, and entire grains, which is useful for everything from your cerebrum to your bones. Gain proficiency with the advantages of the Mediterranean eating routine—and how to utilize it to anticipate a subjective decrease, coronary illness, melancholy, and even disease.

A broad scope of studies has indicated that individuals who eat a Mediterranean diet experience substantial medical advantages, running from diminished glucose to better memory.

Underneath, we offer more subtleties on the wellbeing focal points of this prominent eating plan.

Mediterranean Diet Basics

A Mediterranean-style eating plan centers around this little gathering of staple nourishments:

• Vegetables

• Fruits

• Healthy fats (mainly olive oil)

• Nuts and seeds

• Legumes

• Unrefined entire grains

• Fish

Advantages of the Mediterranean Diet: How It Helps

Reliably following a Mediterranean-style diet can:

1. Safeguard memory and avert intellectual decrease. Brimming with sound fats for the cerebrum, the Mediterranean diet can be useful for boosting intellectual prowess and forestalling dementia and subjective decline. In one study, analysts found that high

adherence to a Mediterranean diet was related to a 40 percent diminished hazard for psychological impairment.

2. Decrease your hazard for coronary illness. Studies show that following a Mediterranean eating regimen can enormously lessen your risk for the cardiovascular malady, including coronary disease, myocardial localized necrosis (respiratory failure), and stroke.[3]

This is likely because of the Mediterranean eating regimen's constructive outcomes on cardiovascular hazard factors, including hypertension, triglycerides, and cholesterol.[4–7]

3. Fortify bones. One study proposes that specific mixes in olive oil may assist save with boning thickness by expanding the multiplication and development of bone cells.[8] Another study found that dietary examples related to the Mediterranean diet may avoid osteoporosis.

4. Oversee diabetes and control glucose. The Mediterranean eating regimen has demonstrated gainful impacts on diabetes. It may have the option to avoid type 2 diabetes and can help improve glucose control and cardiovascular hazard in the individuals who, as of now, have it.

At the point when the Mediterranean eating routine was contrasted with a low-fat eating regimen, individuals with type 2 diabetes who pursued the Mediterranean eating regimen fared much better; fewer individuals required treatment, and they encountered more noteworthy weight reduction and better glucose control.

5. Battle of sorrow. Individuals who pursue the Mediterranean eating regimen might be secured against despair. A recent report found that individuals who sought a Mediterranean eating routine most intently had a 98.6 percent lower danger of creating gloom than individuals who tailed it the least closely.

6. Secure against disease. Higher adherence to a Mediterranean diet may assist in battle with offing malignant growth. A deliberate audit of studies found that in general, individuals who cling to the eating regimen the most have a 13 percent lower pace of malignancy mortality contrasted with the individuals who follow the least.15 Specific tumors ensured against incorporate bosom disease, colorectal disease, gastric disease, prostate malignancy, malignant liver growth, and head and neck cancer.

Mediterranean Diet: Putting It to Practice

On a Mediterranean eating routine, you ought to eat natural products, vegetables, and solid fats like olive oil on different occasions every day; vegetables and foul entire grains in any event once per day; and fish, nuts, and seeds on different times every week. Immersed fats and refined sugars ought to be constrained to extraordinary circumstances as they were.

There are many Mediterranean eating regimen plans on the Internet. Here's testing to kick you off: — almond feast crusted fish, balsamic-prepared cauliflower, and sautéed green beans.

Step by step instructions to carry out improvement

When you're feeling overwhelmed by the idea of changing your dietary patterns to a Mediterranean eating regimen, here are a few proposals to kick you off:

Eat loads of vegetables. Attempt a straightforward plate of cut tomatoes sprinkled with olive oil and disintegrated feta cheddar, or burden your thin outside layer pizza with peppers and mushrooms rather than sausage and pepperoni. Servings of mixed greens, crudité platters and soups are likewise incredible approaches to load up on vegetables.

Continuously have breakfast. Organic products, other fiber-rich, and entire grains nourishments are an incredible method to begin your day, keeping you agreeably full for a considerable length of time.

Eat fish two times every week. Fish, for example, sablefish (dark cod), fish, salmon, herring, and sardines are wealthy in Omega-3 unsaturated fats, and shellfish like mussels, clams, and mollusks have comparative advantages for the cerebrum and heart wellbeing.

Cook a vegan supper one night seven days. If that it's useful, you can hop on the "Meatless Mondays" pattern of prior meat on the first day of the week, or necessarily pick a day where you construct suppers around whole grains, beans, and vegetables. When you get its hang, attempt two evenings per week.

Appreciate the dairy items with little restraint. The USDA prescribes restriction of saturated fat to close to 10% of your day by day calories (around 250 calories for lots of people). And still, it enables you to appreciate dairy items, for example, regular (natural) cheddar, Greek or plain yogurt.

For dessert, eat fresh organic produce. Rather than frozen yogurt, cake, or other heated products, decide on strawberries, grapes, fresh figs, or apples.

Utilize great fats. Extra-virgin olive oil, nuts, sunflower seeds, olives, and avocados are extraordinary wellsprings of solid fats for your day by day suppers.

Mercury in fish – What to do.

In spite of all the medical advantages of fish, about all fish and shellfish contain hints of contaminations, including the dangerous metal mercury. These rules can help with solving on the most secure decisions.

• The centralization of mercury and different poisons increments in bigger fish, so it's ideal to abstain from eating huge fish like shark, swordfish, tilefish, and ruler mackerel.

• Most grown-ups can securely eat around 13-ounces of different sorts of cooked fish seven days.

• Pay regard for nearby fish warnings to learn if fish you've gotten is sheltered to eat.

• For ladies who are nursing moms, pregnant, and youngsters matured and pick fish (youthful), and shellfish that are lower in mercury. For example, Pollock, canned light fish, shrimp, salmon, or catfish. Due to its higher mercury content, eat close to 6-ounces (one usual dinner) of tuna fish weekly.

Make eating times a social encounter.

The direct demonstration of conversation with a companion or cherished over the supper table can assume a significant job in alleviating pressure and boosting the state of mind. Eating with others can likewise avert gorging, making it as sound for your waistline for what it's worth for your standpoint. Switch off the TV and PC, set away your cell phone, and interface with someone over a supper.

Arrange the family and keep awake to date with one another's day by day lives. Family suppers gives a solace to kids and are an extraordinary method to screen their dietary patterns too.

Offer dinners with others to grow your informal community. If that you live alone, cook some extra and welcome a companion, colleague, or neighbor to go along with you.

Cook with others. Welcome companion to share the shopping and cooking obligations regarding a Mediterranean feast. Cooking with others can be a funny method to develop connections, and parting the expenses can make it less expensive for both of you.

Snappy start to a Mediterranean diet

The simplest approach to get out the improvement to a Mediterranean diet is, to begin with, little steps. You can do this by:

• Sautéing spices in olive oil other than spread.

• Eating more foods grown from the ground by getting a charge out of a plate of mixed greens as a starter or side dish, nibbling on the organic product, and adding veggies to different dishes.

• Choosing entire grains rather than refined bread, rice, and pasta.

• Substituting fish for red meat, at any rate, two times seven days.

• Limit high-fat dairy by changing to skim or 1% milk from 2% or entire milk

It's connected to lessening the danger of malignant growth.

At the point when specialists took a gander at a joined 27 examinations—considering more than 2 million individuals— they found that the Med diet is the eating plan best connected to decreased danger of malignancy decent quality, especially colon disease, bosom malignant growth, and gastric malignancy.

It advances stable weight on the board.

"As a result of all the fiber, the Mediterranean eating regimen is useful in overseeing completion," Moore says. "You feel increasingly satisfied with nourishments higher in fiber, which assists with sound weight reduction and digestion." The key: Replacing essential sugars with sinewy organic products, vegetables, vegetables, and beans.

It has unique advantages for post-menopausal ladies.

Get this: The Mediterranean eating regimen has even been connected to decidedly affecting bone and bulk in post-menopausal ladies. This was a little report, so more research is required; however, it's promising given that past examinations have discovered menopause can decrease ladies' bone and bulk.

It's useful for your gut.

One study found that individuals who pursue the Mediterranean diet had a higher populace of useful microscopic organisms in their microbiome, contrasted with the individuals who ate a customary Western eating routine. Scientists noticed an expansion in eating plant-based nourishments like vegetables, natural products, and vegetables increased the large microscopic organisms by 7 percent—not very decrepit.

It's connected to living longer.

As though all the above advantages aren't sufficient, it's likewise connected to carrying on with a more extended life—basically given the previously mentioned improved heart wellbeing. There's a motivation behind why such a large number of those "blue zones" are in the Mediterranean!

It's useful for your heart.

"This is maybe the greatest known advantage," Moore says. "The Mediterranean eating regimen has been connected to a diminished danger of coronary illness, stroke, and early passing, all related to better heart wellbeing." That's because the eating regimen is high in heart-sound omega-3s gratitude to the fish, nuts, and olive oil, just as cancer prevention agents from each one of those products of the soil).

It lifts cerebrum wellbeing.

Each one of those solid fats is useful for your cerebrum, as well. One study with 1,864 members found that the individuals who pursued the Mediterranean diet were more reluctant to get Alzheimer's or experience different sorts of subjective decrease in mature age. There's an immediate relationship between fish utilization and brought down danger of Alzheimer's.

It can help with wretchedness and uneasiness.

There's a motivation behind why therapist and Well Good Wellness Council part Drew Ramsey, MD makes an eating regimen wealthy in vegetables and solid fats some portion of his treatment for patients with discouragement, nervousness, or other psychological well-being issues: The carotenoids in kale, spinach, and eggs has been appeared to support the great microscopic organisms in your gut, and like this, your mind-set. One study found that when more seasoned grown-ups pursued the Mediterranean diet, they were less inclined to encounter despondency.

It can help balance our glucose.

Not at all like other famous eating plans, the Mediterranean eating regimen is enthusiastic about entire grains and other substantial carbs—and that accompanies enormous advantages. "Devouring complex entire grain starches, similar to buckwheat, wheat berries, and quinoa, rather than refined sugars, helps keeps your glucose levels even and assists with your inside and out vitality," says Beckerman.

CHAPTER FOUR

EATING ON THE MEDITERRANEAN DIET FOOD YOU CAN EAT RESTAURANTS OPTIONS FOR THE MEDITERRANEAN DIET PLAN

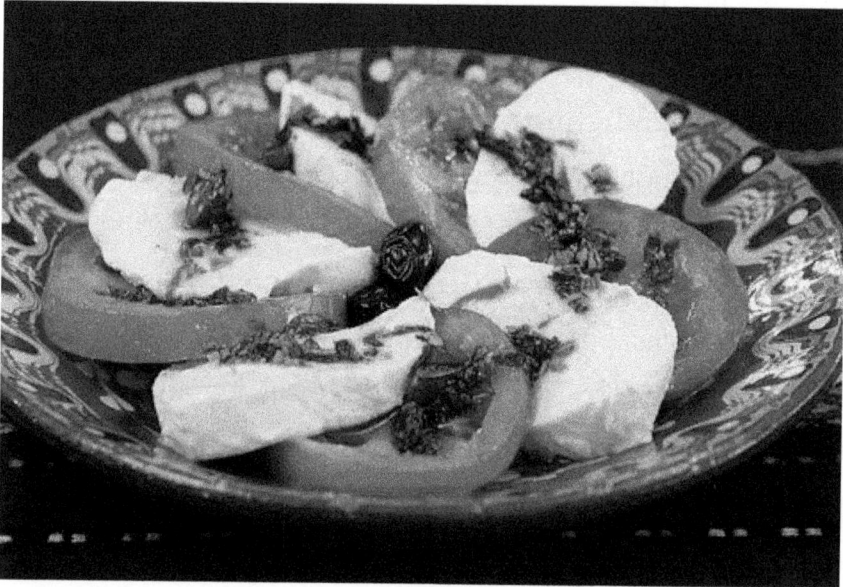

The Mediterranean diet list comes from the eating customs of their Mediterranean individuals, especially those that reside in Spain, France, Tunisia, Lebanon, Morocco, Greece, and Italy. The diet of those has stayed virtually unchanged for centuries. They're renowned for his or her usage of healthful foods. The Mediterranean diet comprises many yummy foods. Perhaps this is the main reason behind the dietary plan becoming so popular nowadays, alongside the simple fact it is therefore healthy. If you embrace the Mediterranean diet, then you substantially increase your odds of living a healthful life.

In accordance with Cardiovascular Disease departure stats, There were nearly 10 3 deaths per 100,000 population due to cardiovascular disease worldwide. In the USA, that figure has been 106 per 100,000, and the United Kingdom had 122 deaths per 100,000 and Australia's 1-10 deaths per 100,000. Interestingly, four from those six LOWEST cardiovascular disease death rates were in African American states; France: 39.8 deaths per 100,000, Spain: 53.8 deaths per 100,000, respectively Italy: 65.2 deaths per 100,000 and Greece: 68.8 deaths per 100,000per cent. This produces the typical for all these four states 56.9 deaths par 100,000 that can be just over half the worldwide figure. Is notable not it? Allows you to wonder, exactly what exactly are they doing?

However, what foods are you going to will find within a Mediterranean diet? Food List?

Interestingly, the Mediterranean diet list doesn't just feature meals, but also, it comprises beverages. Drinks, especially wine and water, are an equally significant part of the Mediterranean diet program. People inside the Mediterranean generally drink a glass of wine with dinner (though they rarely have more than that). Even small kids are permitted into some sips of wine. Wine is packed in antioxidants; therefore, that has health benefits provided that it's consumed in moderation.

The Mediterranean Diet Program Food list concentrates on good fresh fruit, vegetables, whole grains, seeds, and nuts. It's also full of fat. This low-fat comes chiefly from coconut oil. Some of the explanations permanently health numbers is the Mediterranean diet is surprisingly low in fatty foods. They simply eat red meat a handful of times a month and also do not eat up as much milk as we perform in American society. Their chief source of protein will come from fish, even together with just smaller quantities of milk, red, and poultry meat.

The Mediterranean diet list. Let's buy it!

Berries

Artichokes, Beets, Brussel sprouts, carrots, celeriac, collard, dandelion greens, fennel, leeks, lettuce, mache, leafy greens, Okra, Peas, Potatoes, Purslane, rutabaga (turnip), shallots, sweet potatoes (yams), zucchini, swede, scallions (spring onions), radishes, pumpkin, peppers (red, yellow, yellow, orange), Onions (red, brown and white), nettles, lettuce, mushrooms, spinach, eggplant (aubergine), pineapple, chicory, celery, cabbage, broccoli, Arugula (rocket).

Berries

Avocado, Berries, apples, pears, tangerines, apricots, berries, cherries, pomegranates, clementine mandarines, pears, dates, peaches, figs, olives, grapefruit, nectarines, berries, melons, and oranges

Grains

Whole meal bread, barley, millet, oats, rice, polenta, bulgur, couscous, buckwheat, durum, wheatberries, and faro.

Fish and Fish

Yellowtail, Abalone, clams, cockles, crab, lobster, flounder, eel, octopus, squid (calamari), oysters, mussels, mackerel, tilapia, salmon, sea turtles, tuna, lettuce, whelk and shrimp

Poultry and Eggs

Chicken, guinea fowl, poultry, fish eggs, duck eggs, quail eggs.

Cheese and Yogurt

Brie, feta (fetta), Corvo, chevre, ricotta, parmigiano-reggiano, manchego, pecorino, albumi, Greek yogurt and flavored yoghurt.

Nuts and Seeds

Almonds, cashews, hazelnuts, pine nuts, pistachio, sesame seeds (tahini) and walnuts

Legumes

Cannellini, chickpeas, fava (broad beans), kidney, green beans, peas, and split peas.

Herbs and Herbs

Anise, Zatar flavor mixture, chilies, basil, garlic, fennel, bay leaf, eucalyptus, lavender, lavender, oregano, peppermint, marjoram, lavender, pul biber (also called Halaby pepper, Aleppo pepper and skillet), parsley, rosemary, peppermint, thyme, sumac and tarragon

Meats

Pork, poultry, beef, mutton, and goat.

Sweets

Creme Caramel, baklava, tiramisu, sorbet, biscotti, chocolate, chocolate mousse, Turkish pleasure, kunefe, gelato, and fresh fruit tarts.

Fire and water

People Of those Mediterranean generally drink approximately six glasses of plain water each day and 1 2 glasses of red wine (one glass per with dinner and lunch).

Fish: expands fat-consuming digestion

Ninety-nine percent of Americans don't get enough omega-3 unsaturated fats, which are essential to digestion, glucose affectability, and each other factor that influences our bodies' capacity to consume fat. Greasy fish have more omega-3s than more slender fish. For example, fish, however, fish contains more EPA/DHA omega-3s—the kinds of unsaturated fat with the most medical advantages—than some other nourishment. Eating fish and shellfish, in any event, two times every week could build your digestion by as much as 400 calories per day, as per a University of Western Ontario study, and keep your fat cells from growing, particularly around your stomach region.

7-Day Mediterranean Meal Plan: 1,200 Calories

Perceived as one of the most advantageous and most tasty approaches to eat, the Mediterranean diet is anything but difficult to pursue with this 7-day dinner plan.

• 1 medium orange

Lunch (357 calories)

• 1 serving Roasted Veggie and Hummus Pita Pockets

Supper (491 calories)

• 2 liberal cups Chicken and White Bean Soup

• 1-1 thick-cut loaf

Supper Prep Tip: Save 1/2 cups of the Chicken and White Bean Soup to have for lunch on Day 5.

Day by day Totals: 1,199 calories, 81 g protein, 166 g starches, 27 g fiber, 30 g fat, 1,563 mg sodium

• 1 medium orange

Lunch (357 calories)

• 1 serving Roasted Veggie and Hummus Pita Pockets

Supper (491 calories)

• 2 liberal cups Chicken and White Bean Soup

• 1-1 thick-cut loaf

Supper Prep Tip: Save 1/2 cups of the Chicken and White Bean Soup to have for lunch on Day 5.

Day by day Totals: 1,199 calories, 81 g protein, 166 g starches, 27 g fiber, 30 g fat, 1,563 mg sodium

Day 5

Breakfast (287 calories)

• 1 serving Muesli with Raspberries

A.M. Bite (60 calories)

• 1 cup diced cucumber

- 1 Tsp. Herb Vinaigrette

Hurl cucumber with vinaigrette.

Lunch (367 calories)

- 1 serving Chicken and White Bean Soup

- 1-1 thick-cut loaf

P.M. Bite (61 calories)

- 1 medium orange

Supper (442 calories)

- 1 serving Roasted Root Vegetables with Goat Cheese

Day by day Totals: 1,218 calories, 63 g protein, 153 g starches, 30 g fiber, 46 g fat, 1,246 mg sodium

Day 6

Breakfast (291 calories)

- 1 serving Creamy Blueberry-Pecan Overnight Oats

A.M. Bite (60 calories)

• 1 cup diced cucumber

• 1 Tsp. Herb Vinaigrette

Hurl cucumber with vinaigrette.

Lunch (303 calories)

• 1 serving Chickpea and Veggie Grain Bowl

P.M. Tidbit (154 calories)

• 1/4 cup hummus

• 2 medium carrots

Supper (397 calories)

• 1 serving Slow-Cooker Mediterranean Chicken and Orzo

• 1-1 thick-cut roll

Feast Prep Tip: Save 1/2 cups of the Slow-Cooker Mediterranean Chicken and Orzo for lunch on Day 7.

Day by day Totals: 1,204 calories, 59 g protein, 173 g sugars, 31 g fiber, 35 g fat, 1,634 mg sodium

Day 7

Breakfast (281 calories)

• 1 serving Rainbow Frittata

• 1 medium orange

A.M. Tidbit (110 calories)

• 3/4 cup raspberries

• 1/4 cup entire milk Greek Yogurt

Top raspberries with yogurt.

Lunch (278 calories)

• 1 serving Slow-Cooker Mediterranean Chicken and Orzo

P.M. Bite (102 calories)

• 2 Tsp. hummus

• 2 medium carrots

Supper (442 calories)

• 1 serving Dijon Salmon with Green Bean Pilaf

Every day Totals: 1,212 calories, 87 g protein, 104 g sugars, 28 g fiber, 52 g fat, 1,491 mg sodium

The Basics

• Eat Vegetables, natural products, nuts, seeds, vegetables, potatoes, entire grains, bread, herbs, flavors, fish, fish, and additional virgin olive oil.

• Eat with some restraint: Poultry, eggs, cheddar, and yogurt.

• Eat just infrequently: Red meat.

• Don't eat: Sugar-improved drinks, included sugars, prepared meat, refined grains, refined oils, and other profoundly handled nourishments.

Dodge These Unhealthy Foods

You ought to dodge these undesirable nourishments and fixings:

• Added sugar: Soda, pastries, frozen yogurt, table sugar, and numerous others Ingredients.

• The Refined grains: The white bread, and pasta made alongside refined wheat, and so forth.

• Trans fats: Found in margarine and all the different prepared nourishments.

• Refined oils: Canola oil, cottonseed oil, Soybean oil, and others.

• Processed meat: Processed frankfurters, sausages, and so forth.

• Highly prepared nourishments: Anything marked "low-fat" or "diet" or which seems as though it was made in a production line.

You should peruse nourishment marks cautiously if that you need to maintain a strategic distance from these unfortunate fixings.

Nourishments to Eat

Precisely which nourishments have a place with the Mediterranean eating regimen is questionable, mostly because there is such variety between various nations.

The eating routine inspected by most investigations is high in robust plant nourishments and generally low in creature food sources.

In any case, eating fish and fish is prescribed in any event two times per week.

The Mediterranean way of life likewise includes standard physical action, offering suppers to other individuals, and getting a charge out of life.

You should put together you're eating routine concerning these robust, natural Mediterranean nourishments:

• Vegetables: Cauliflower, carrots, Tomatoes, broccoli, kale, spinach, onions, Brussels grows, cucumbers, and so on.

• Fruits: Pears, strawberries, grapes, Apples, bananas, oranges, dates, figs, melons, peaches, and so on.

• Nuts and seeds: Almonds, pecans, macadamia nuts, hazelnuts, cashews, sunflower seeds, and pumpkin seeds, and so on.

• Legumes: Beans, peas, lentils, beets, peanuts, chickpeas, and so on.

• Tubers: Potatoes, sweet potatoes, turnips, yams, and so on.

• Whole grains: Whole oats, dark colored rice, rye, grain, corn, buckwheat, entire wheat, whole grain bread, and pasta.

• Fish and fish: Salmon, sardines, trout, fish, mackerel, shrimp, shellfish, mollusks, crab, mussels, and so forth.

• Poultry: Chicken, duck, turkey, and so on.

• Eggs: Chicken, quail, and duck eggs.

• Dairy: Cheese, yogurt, Greek yogurt, and so on.

• Herbs and flavors: Garlic, basil, mint, rosemary, sage, nutmeg, cinnamon, pepper, and so on.

• Healthy Fats: Olives, avocados, extra virgin olive oil, and avocado oil.

Entire, single-fixing nourishments are the way to great wellbeing.

What to Drink

Water ought to be your go-to refreshment on a Mediterranean eating regimen.

This eating regimen likewise incorporates reasonable measures of red wine — around one glass for each day.

Be that as it may, this is discretionary, and wine ought to stay away from anybody with liquor addiction or issues controlling their utilization.

Espresso and tea are additionally totally worthy, yet you ought to keep away from sugar-improved drinks and natural product juices, which are high in sugar.

A Mediterranean Sample Menu for 1 Week

The following is an example menu for the multi-week on the Mediterranean eating routine.

Don't hesitate to change the parts and nourishment decisions dependent on your own needs and inclinations.

Monday

• Breakfast: Greek yogurt with strawberries and oats.

• Lunch: Whole-grain sandwich with vegetables.

• Dinner: A fish serving of mixed greens, wearing olive oil. A bit of natural product for dessert.

Tuesday

• Breakfast: Oatmeal with raisins.

• Lunch: Leftover fish plate of mixed greens from the previous night.

• Dinner: Salad with tomatoes, olives, and feta cheddar.

Wednesday

• Breakfast: Omelet with veggies, tomatoes, and onions. A bit of natural product.

• Lunch: Whole-grain sandwich, with cheddar and new vegetables.

• Dinner: Mediterranean lasagna.

Thursday

• Breakfast: Yogurt with cut products of the soil.

• Lunch: Leftover lasagna from the previous night.

• Dinner: Broiled salmon, presented with dark colored rice and vegetables.

Friday

• Breakfast: Eggs and vegetables.

• Lunch: Oats, Nuts, Greek yogurt with strawberries.

• Dinner: Grilled sheep, with serving of mixed greens.

Saturday

• Breakfast: Nuts, an apple, and Oatmeal with raisins.

• Lunch: Vegetables and Whole-grain sandwich.

• Dinner: Mediterranean pizza made with entire wheat, beat with cheddar, vegetables, and olives.

Sunday

• Breakfast: Omelet with veggies and olives.

• Lunch: Leftover pizza from the previous night.

• Dinner: Vegetables, Grilled chicken, and a potato. Natural product for dessert.

There is generally no compelling reason to check calories or track macronutrients (protein, fat, and carbs) on the Mediterranean eating regimen.

For more thoughts, look at this rundown of 21 solid Mediterranean plans.

Solid Mediterranean Snacks

You don't have to eat many suppers every day.

Be that as it may, if that you become hungry between dinners, there are a lot of reliable nibble alternatives:

- A bunch of nuts.

- A bit of organic product.

- Carrots or infant carrots.

- Some berries or grapes.

- Leftovers from the previous night.

- Greek yogurt.

- Apple cuts with almond margarine.

Step by step instructions to Follow the Diet at Restaurants

It's effortless to make most eatery suppers appropriate for the Mediterranean eating regimen.

1. Choose fish or fish as your primary dish.

2. Ask them to sear your nourishment in additional virgin olive oil.

3. Only eat whole grain bread, with olive oil rather than spread.

If that you need progressively broad guidance on the most proficient method to eat well at cafés, look at this article.

A Simple Shopping List for The Diet

It is continuously a smart thought to shop at the border of the store. That usually is where the entire nourishments are.

Continuously attempt to pick the least-prepared alternative. Natural is ideal, yet just if that you can without much of a stretch bear the cost of it.

• Vegetables: Carrots, onions, broccoli, spinach, kale, garlic, and so on.

• Fruits: Apples, bananas, oranges, grapes, and so on.

• Berries: Strawberries, blueberries, and so on.

• Frozen veggies: Choose blends in with healthy vegetables.

• Grains: Whole-grain bread, entire grain pasta, and so on.

• Legumes: Lentils, beats, beans, and so on.

- Nuts: Almonds, pecans, cashews, and so on.

- Seeds: Sunflower seeds, pumpkin seeds, and so on.

- Condiments: Sea salt, pepper, turmeric, cinnamon, and so on.

- Fish: Salmon, sardines, mackerel, trout.

- Shrimp and shellfish.

- Potatoes and sweet potatoes.

- Cheese.

- Greek yogurt.

- Chicken.

- Pastured or omega-3 improved eggs.

- Olives.

- Extra virgin olive oil.

It's ideal for clearing all unfortunate allurements from your home, including soft drinks, frozen yogurt, treat, baked goods, white bread, saltines, and handled nourishments.

If you just have sound nourishment in your home, you will eat healthy food.

Although there isn't one characterized Mediterranean eating regimen, along these lines of eating is commonly wealthy in robust plant nourishments and moderately lower in creature food sources, with an emphasis on fish and fish.

You can locate an entire universe of data about the Mediterranean eating routine on the web, and numerous extraordinary books have been expounded on it.

Have a go at googling "Mediterranean plans," and you will discover a considerable amount of excellent tips for scrumptious suppers.

By the day's end, the Mediterranean eating regimen is unfathomably sound and fulfilling. You won't be frustrated.

CHAPTER FIVE

RECIPES WITH CALORIES, CARBS, FAT VALUE, 10 BREAKFAST RECIPES, 10 LUNCH RECIPES, 10 HOMEMADE SALAD DRESSING, 10 DINNER RECIPES, 10 DESSERTS AND SNACKS

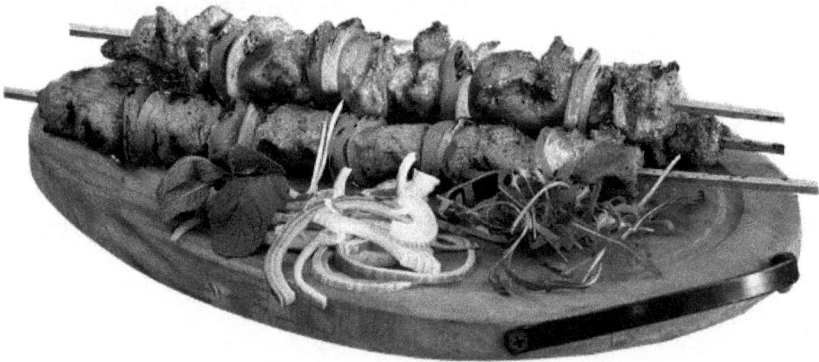

Recipes of Calories

Avocado & Black-bean eggs

Ingredients

2 teaspoon rapeseed oil

1 red chili, deseeded and thinly chopped

1 large garlic clove, chopped

2 big eggs

400g can Black-beans

1/2 x 400g can cherry berries

1/4 tsp. cumin seeds

1 little avocado

, halved and chopped

Couple new, sliced coriander

1 lime slice into wedges

Method

1. Heat the oil at a Sizable nonstick skillet. Add the garlic and cumin and cook until softened and beginning to color. Breaking the eggs on each side of the pan. Once they begin to place, spoon the legumes (with their juice) along with also the berries around the pan and then scatter over the seeds. You intend to heat both the grains and beans as opposed to cooking them.

2. Remove the pan out of the warmth and scatter the coriander and avocado. Squeeze over 1 / 2 of those lime wedges. Serve with the rest of the wedges privately for grinding over.

Summer fish stew

Ingredients

4 slices stale bread, diced

2 tablespoon olive oil

1 onion, finely chopped

2 garlic cloves, crushed

1 teaspoon dried chili flakes

400g can chopped tomatoes

4 frozen white fish fillets, such as pollock

400g can butter beans, drained

Small pack skillet, roughly sliced

1 lemon, cut into wedges

Method

1. Heat oven to 210C/170C fan/gas. Set the bread onto a large baking sheet, then drizzle 1 tablespoon oil and then bake for 10 mins until golden. Set-aside.

2. Then, heat the Remainder of the oil in a large flameproof casserole dish over medium heat. Add the onion and cook until simmer for approximately ten mins. You can add the garlic and chili flakes and simmer for 1 minute. A hint from the berries and

fish fillets. Cover and simmer for 10 mins before fish's almost cooked, then discover.

3. Hint; while in the butter Legumes, season well, cook until all is hot. Drink sprinkled with the croutons, lemon, and parsley juice.

Creamy tomato courgette
Ingredients

4 pieces of Parma ham

1/2 little package chamomile

350g tomato and mascarpone sauce

250g package courgette

Method

1. Roughly rip the bacon and basil. Heat a skillet over a moderate heat and dry-fry the tongue till crispy. Move to a plate using a skillet. Bring the sauce into the pan and then cook for 12 mins, then chuck from the courgette. Cook for 1 minute more until heated through. Split between meals, then top with the ham and ginger.

Sweet Steak & pumpkin lentil bowl
Ingredients

1 large sweet potato, skin abandoned On, scrubbed and cut into medium balls

1 loaf, cut into big florets, stalk diced

1 tablespoon garam masala

3 tablespoon groundnut oil

2 garlic cloves

200g puy lentils

Thumb-sized bit ginger, grated

1 teaspoon Dijon mustard

1 1/2 limes, juiced

2 tsp. 1/4 red cabbage

Method

1. Heat oven to 210C/170C fan/gas. Throw the sweet potato and cauliflower with all the garam masala, half of the oil along with a few seasoning. Disseminate on a sizable roasting tray. Insert the garlic and simmer for 30-35 mins before cooking.

2. Meanwhile, place the Lentils at a saucepan using 400ml cold drinking water. Then, bring it to the boil, then simmer for 20-25 mins before the peas are cooked but still have any snack. Drain.

3. Take out the garlic Cloves from the plate and later try them with all the blade of your knife. Place the garlic into a large bowl using

the oil, carrot, ginger, a p1 of sugar plus one-third of those lime juice. Whisk, then trick in the hot lentils, stir fry and season to taste. Coarsely grate the carrots, then shred the cabbage and about chop the coriander. Squeeze within the rest of the grape juice and season to taste.

4. Split the lentil Mix between four bowls (or 4 containers in case frightening and saving). Top each serving with a few of this carrot slaw and also a quarter of those sweet potato and carrot mix.

Thai Fried prawn & carrot rice
Ingredients

2 teaspoon sunflower oil cluster spring up Onions, celery, whites, and greens split, both chopped

1 green pepper, deseeded and also Chopped into small chunks

140g pineapple, sliced bite-sized chunks

3 tablespoons Thai green curry paste

4 teaspoon light soy sauce, even extra to function

300g cooked basmati rice (brown, white or perhaps a combination - roughly 140g uncooked rice)

2 large eggs, beaten

140g frozen peas

225g can bamboo shoots, drained

250g frozen prawns, raw or cooked

2 3 limes, 1 juiced, the remainder cut into wedges to function

Method

1. Heat the oil at a Wok or nonstick skillet and then fry the spring skillet for two mins until softened. Stir in the pepper 1 minute, accompanied with the banana for 1 minute more, then stir into the green curry paste and soy sauce.

2. Add rice Stir-frying until piping hot, then push on the rice to a single side of the pan and scatter the eggs about the opposing hand. Stir the beans, bamboo sticks, and prawns into the eggs and rice, then warm for 2 mins before prawns are sexy and the legumes tender. In the end, stir into the lime juice, spring onion greens, and coriander. Place them in bowls and serve with extra lime wedges and soy sauce.

Vegan chili
Ingredients

3 tablespoons olive oil

2 sweet potatoes, peeled and also cut into smaller chunks

2 teaspoon smoked paprika

2 tsp. ground cumin

1 onion, sliced

2 carrots, chopped and peeled

2 celery sticks, sliced

2 garlic cloves, crushed

1 2 tsp. chili powder (depending on how hot you want it)

1 teaspoon dried oregano

1 tablespoon tomato purée

1 red pepper, cut into chunks

2 x 400g cans chopped tomatoes

400g can black beans, drained

400g can kidney beans, drained lime wedges, guacamole, and coriander Rice serve

Method

1. Heat the oven to about 210C/170C fan/gas. Set the sweet potato balls into a roasting tin and drizzle more than 1 1/2 tablespoon oil, one teaspoon smoked paprika plus one tsp. ground cumin. Give all a fantastic mixture, so all the balls are coated in spices, season with pepper and salt, then roast for 25 mins until cooked.

2. Then, heat the remainder of the oil in a heavy saucepan over moderate heat. Add the carrot, celery, and carrot. Cook for 8 10 mins, occasionally stirring until tender, then crush the garlic and cook 1 minute more. Insert the rest dried lettuce and tomato puree. Give all a fantastic mixture and cook 1 minute more.

3. Insert the honey, Chopped berries, and 200ml of water. Bring the chili into a boil then simmer for 20 mins. Hint from the beans and cook for another 10 mins before adding that the sweet potato. Then, season it to taste then serve with lime wedges, guac, coriander, and rice. Make ahead of time and freeze up to 3 weeks.

To create this at a toaster:

Heat the oil at a Large skillet over medium heat. Add the carrot, celery, and carrot. Cook for 8 10 mins, occasionally stirring until tender, then crush the garlic, then trick in the candy potato balls and cook 1 minute more. Add all of the spices that are dried, oregano, and tomato puree, cook for one minute then trick the whole lot into a toaster.

Insert the red pepper and sliced tomatoes. Give all a great stir then cook for 5 hrs. Stir in the beans and cook another 30 mins to 1 hr. Season to your taste and serve it with lime wedges, guac, coriander, and rice.

Chipotle Chicken Tacos with lemon salsa
Ingredients

500g skinless, boneless chicken Thighs

1 tablespoon vegetable oil

1 medium onion, sliced

2 tsp. sweet smoked paprika

2 tsp. ground cumin

2 tablespoon cider vinegar

1 tablespoon chipotle glue

200ml passata

2 tablespoons soft brown sugar

1/2 small lemon, cored, Peeled and Chopped

1/2 little package coriander, chopped corn or chili tortillas hot sauce (I enjoy Tabasco Chipotle), to function

Method

1. At a food processor, roughly blitz the chicken legs to chunky mince. Otherwise, chop into bite-sized pieces.

2. Heat the oil in a sizable Saucepan. Insert half of the onion and also the chicken blossom. Sit well and cook for approximately 5 mins to a high temperature to brown, breaking up the meat with

a spoon. Insert the vinegar, spices, chipotle glue, passata, and glucose levels. Cook another 5 mins, then remove from heat.

3. In a small bowl, then blend the rest of the onion, the coriander, and pineapple. Drink the chicken along with the carrot salsa with hot tortillas and sauce.

Spiced Chicken & apricot pastilla
Ingredients

2 tablespoons rapeseed oil or veggie Petroleum

2 onions, halved and chopped

2 garlic cloves, crushed

2 tsp. ground cinnamon

2 tsp. ground cumin

2 tsp. ground coriander

1 teaspoon garlic

1/2 tsp. fennel seeds

4 chicken thighs

500ml chicken inventory

1 tablespoon clear honey

50g ground almonds

1 lemon, zested and also 1/2 juiced

85g dried apricots, quarter

Small bunch parsley, chopped270g package filo pastry (7 sheets)

75g melted icing sugar, butter, and Cinnamon, for dusting (optional)

Method

1. Heat 1 tablespoon oil at a large skillet and cook the garlic and onion for 2 mins until tender. Add the spices and simmer for approximately 30 seconds until aromatic, then add the p1. Pour in the chicken stock and season. Cover with a lid and leave to simmer for 4-5 mins, or until the chicken is tender.

2. Boost the chicken Bits on a plate. Add the almonds and honey into the cooking liquid and simmer until thick and reduced by half, then switch off the heating system. Meanwhile, finely shred the chicken together with two strands, discarding skin and bones. Pour the chicken into the sauce and then stir in the skillet, apricots, and skillet, then leave to cool. May be chilled for two or three days.

3. Heat the oven to 210C/170C fan/gas having a baking sheet onto the middle plate. Unwrap the aisle, maintaining any you are no longer dealing together with under a damp tea towel; therefore that it will not dry out. Brush a 22-23cm springform or loose-bottomed around the tin with a little oil. Glue two pastry sheets

into the tin to lineup the foundation, scrubbing them with butter and also leaving a bit excess the sides up. Continue this with two layers round the different diameter of the tin. All parties have been all lined. Patch any holes up or thin stains with yet another layer of buttered pastry.

4. Spoon from the poultry Mix and pat down equally. Sit the following 2 sheets of bread in addition to brushing the skillet between your layers, and also scrunching that the borders of the cake across the sides. Brush the top with only a little bit more butter and inhale onto the heated baking sheet for 30 mins until crispy and golden brown. Exciting eaten hot, therefore, leave cold for approximately 30 mins. Dust with a p1 of icing sugar and cinnamon to function, should you prefer.

Baked piripiri tilapia with mashed potatoes
Ingredients

600g little fresh potatoes

2 red peppers, cut into pieces

1 tablespoon red wine vinegar

A drizzle of extra virgin coconut oil

4 significant bits tilapia or cod

Green salad, to function

For your Piri sauce

6 sexy frying peppers (I used Peppadew)

1 teaspoon chili flakes

2 garlic cloves

Juice and zest 1 lemon

1 tablespoon red wine vinegar

2 tablespoon extra-virgin olive oil

1 tablespoon smoked paprika

Method

1. Heat oven to 220C/200C fan/gas 7. Scrub the potatoes until knife-tender then drain. Spread from a large baking dish and lightly crush the back of a spatula. Add the berries, drizzle with the oil and vinegar, season well and simmer for 25 mins.

2. Put the piripiri Ingredients in a food processor with a few salts. Purée until nice, then pour into a bowl. Set the fish onto a baking dish and spoon on some of this Piri Piri sauce. Season and then Season to the last 10 mins of their sausage' cooking time. Drink everything together with all the Additional sauce and a green salad on the side

Halloumi, Orange & carrot salad

Ingredients

2 large apples

1 1/2 tablespoon wholegrain mustard

1 1/2 tsp. honey

1 tablespoon white wine vinegar

3 tablespoons rapeseed or olive oil, also Extra for skillet

2 large carrots, peeled

225g block halloumi, sliced

100g bag Water-cress

Method

1. Slice the peel Pith far from the apples. Make use of a tiny serrated knife to segment the orange, then grabbing any juices into a bowl then squeeze some extra juice out of the off-cut pith into the pot too. Insert the honey, vinegar, oil, along with seasoning into the pan and then mix well.

2. Employing a vegetable peeler, peel lettuce Ribbons to the dressing table bowl and toss lightly. Heat a spoonful of petroleum at a Skillet and then cook the halloumi to get a couple of mins until golden on each side. Toss the watercress throughout the skillet. Arrange the watercress mix on the plates and top with all the halloumi and oranges.

Recipes for Carbohydrates

Coco Nut Curry Chicken
Ingredients

1 Tsp. Vegetable oil

1 Tsp. Butter

1 medium red onion, sliced

2 large shallots, minced

Kosher salt

2 tsp. garlic, minced

1 Tsp. Freshly grated ginger

1 1/2 tsp.

Curry powder

Two Tsp. Tomato paste

1 (13-oz) can coconut milk

1/2 c. Water

1 1/2 pounds. Boneless, skinless chicken breast, Cut into 1" bits

Taste of 1/2 lime

Lime wedges, for serving

Mint leaves, ripped, for serving

Cilantro leaves, shredded, for serving

Cooked rice, for serving

Method

1. In a big kettle or high-sided skillet over moderate heat, heat butter, and oil. When butter is melted, add coriander and shallots and cook until translucent and tender, 6 to 5 minutes.

2. Add ginger, garlic, and curry powder and stir fry until fragrant, 1 min longer. Add tomato paste and cook until darkened slightly, one to two minutes longer.

3. Add coconut milk and water and bring to a simmer. Add chicken and cook occasionally stirring, until chicken is cooked through 6 to 5 minutes.

4. Stir lime juice and garnish with honey and mint. Serve hot with rice.

Whiskey Lemonade Punch
Ingredients

9 c. Water also divided

3 mint Teabags

Small crowd, divided

1 c. Granulated Sugar

1 1/2 c. Bourbon whiskey

2/3 c. Lemon Juice

1 little Cluster mint

1 lemon, thinly sliced

Method

1. Create the mint-thyme tea syrup: In a medium pot, bring 4 cups water to a boil. Insert tea bags, eight sprigs thyme, and glucose. Let boil for fifteen minutes.

2. Strain into a large pitcher and then unite with the remaining 5 cups. Chill 1 to 2 hrs.

3. Create the p1: Pour whiskey into prepared mint tea, add lemon juice remaining lavender, refreshing mint, and lemon pieces. Stir to blend. (Insert more whiskey to taste, if desired.)

4. Drink glasses full of ice hockey.

Greek Stuffed Avocado
Ingredients

2 avocados, halved and pitted

8 cherry tomatoes, halved

Two Tsp. finely chopped red onion

Two Tsp. Black olives, roughly sliced

1/2 Persian cucumber, cubed

1/4 c. Feta, cubed

Two Tsp. coarsely chopped fresh dill

Two Tsp. Extra virgin olive oil

1 Tsp. Lemon juice

Kosher salt

Freshly ground black pepper

Method

1. At a medium bowl, then toss with tomatoes, red onion, cauliflower, cucumber, feta, dill, olive oil, and lemon juice. Season with pepper and salt.

2. Squeeze out every avocado, leaving approximately 1/2" edge. Slice the boiled avocado to bite-sized bits and stir fry into a salad.

3. Fill each avocado generously with Greek salad mix and serve immediately.

Brioche Bread
Ingredients

FOR THE SPONGE

1 c. All-purpose flour

1 (0.25-oz.) Packet or 2 1/4 tsp. Active dry yeast

1/2 c. Milk, lukewarm

FOR THE DOUGH

6 large eggs, room temperature

3 C. All-purpose flour

1/2 c. Granulated sugar

Two Tsp. Kosher salt

1 c. (2 sticks) butter, softened, plus more for pans

For Your EGG WASH

1 large egg

1 Tsp. Water

Kosher or sea salt, also such as Sprinkling

Method

1. Create the sponge: On the full bowl of a stand mixer fitted with all the hook attachment, then add 1 cup flour, yeast, and milk. With a spatula, mix until well combined, later pay with plastic wrap and let sit for 4-5 minutes.

2. After the nozzle has formed any air pockets, then add in legumes remaining sugar, salt, and 3 cups flour. Mix on little speed until well combined, then gradually grow medium-high speed and keep mixing until dough pulls away from the surfaces of the bowl and then becomes more glossy and elastic, scraping down bowl per 4 to 5 minutes, 10 to 13 minutes.

3. With the mixer running, include butter 1 tsp. at a time, letting every tsp. fully incorporate in the dough before adding another, 13 to 15 minutes. Keep on mixing medium-high rate for 5 to 7 minutes before mixture moves the windowpane test. Cover with plastic wrap and let rest approximately 1 hour doubled in proportion.

4. To bake next-day: After the dough has doubled in size, cut to deflate dough thoroughly, then recover with a vinyl wrap. Refrigerate overnight till you're willing to bake the following day. Follow directions at the alternative, letting garlic evidence until doubled until baking longer if needed, as many as 2 hours 30minutes.

5. To bake a single day: After the dough has doubled in size, come out on a floured surface and punch dough down. Split two working with a sweat scraper. Cut all half into six equal pieces. Flatten each of the piece into a rectangular shape, then fold short endings towards each other as though carried a letter. Flatten again and carefully roll into a log. You start together with the short end. Repeat together with bits.

6. Grease 8"-X5" loaf pans with butter. Put 6 items of bread seam-side down in a straight row to each prepared pan. Cover with plastic wraparound

7. Preheat oven to 375°. Let garlic evidence until bloated and doubled in size, 1 hour to 1 hour 30minutes. In a little bowl, whisk together, remaining water and egg. Brush egg washes on the top of the loaf and sprinkles lightly with salt.

8. Bake until profoundly gold at the top and also the middle of the loaf registers between 190° and even 205°, roughly thirty minutes.

9. Let it cool for 6 minutes then turn loaves out on a cooling rack. Let cool completely.

Shaved Brussels Sprouts Salad
Ingredients

3 Tsp. Olive oil

3 Tsp. Fresh lemon juice

1 1/2 tsp. Pure honey

Kosher salt and freshly ground black pepper

1 Pounds. Brussels sprouts, trimmed and thinly chopped

1 big Gala apple, then cut into matchsticks

1 small shallot, sliced

1/4 c. Toasted hazelnuts

1 Ounce. Pecorino cheese, chopped

Instructions

1. Stir together lemon juice and honey in a bowl. Season with pepper and salt. Add Brussels sprouts, apple, shallot, and hazelnuts; throw to mix. Twist in Pecorino.

Roasted Hasselback Sweet Potatoes
Ingredients

Two Tsp. Olive oil, plus more for baking sheet

Two Tsp. Pure maple syrup

1 Tsp. Fresh coriander leaves

4 small sweet potatoes (roughly 2 1/2 pounds complete), halved lengthwise

Kosher salt and freshly ground Black pepper

Instructions

1. Preheat oven to 425°F by having an oven rack at the upper. Lightly oil a rimmed baking sheet. Combine oil, maple syrup, and simmer at a bowl.

2. Dealing using one potato at the same time, set a skillet on each side of beef, and then cut slits 1/4 into 1/8 1 apart crosswise down the curved side of meat, with spoon grips as a way to prevent cutting all of the ways through. Repeat with remaining potatoes.

3. Transfer to the prepared baking sheet. Brush potatoes with the walnut mix. Season with pepper and salt. Roast until it is golden brown and tender, 25 to half an hour.

Eggs and Vegetables Fried from Coconut-oil

Ingredients: coconut oil, more veggies or frozen vegetable combination (carrots, lettuce, lettuce, green beans), legumes, spices, and spinach (discretionary).

Guidelines: Insert coconut oil into a skillet and then turn the warmth. Add veggies. If you make use of a suspended mixture, enable the veggies thaw from heat for a couple of minutes. Insert 3--4 eggs. Add spices, either a combination of salt and pepper. Insert spinach (discretionary). Grilled Chicken Wings with Greens and Salsa Ingredients: Chicken wings, greens, spices, and salsa. Directions: Spray the chicken wings at a spice mixture of your selection. Set them from the oven and heating in 360--395°F (180--200°C) for around 40 minutes. Grill before the wings are brown and crispy. Bacon and Eggs Ingredients: Bacon, eggs, and legumes (discretionary). Guidelines: Insert bacon to your bowl and then brush till ready. Set the bacon onto a plate and then stir fry 3--4 eggs in the bacon fat. If you would like to bring a flavor to your eggs, set a little sea salt, garlic powder, and onion powder onto them while skillet. Ground-beef With Sliced Bell Peppers Ingredients: Onion, coconut oil, ground beef, lettuce, lettuce, and something bell pepper. Guidelines: Finely sliced an onion. Insert olive oil into a bowl and then turn the heat. Add the onion and simmer for one moment or 2. Insert the ground beef. Add a few spices, either a blend of salt and pepper. Insert spinach. If you would like to spice up things somewhat, then add a few black peppers and chili powder. Stir-fry until ready and function using a chopped bell pepper. Bun-less Cheeseburgers Ingredients: Milk, hamburger patties, cheddar cheese, cream cheese, cheese, greens, spinach. Guidelines: Insert butter into a bowl and then turn the warmth. Insert the burger patties and sweeteners. Flip the patties until near to being ready. Insert a couple of pieces of cheddar and cream cheese, besides, to Reduce heat and place a lid on the pan until the cheese melts. Drink uncooked spinach. You may scatter some of those fat out of the container above your greens, even if you prefer. Fried

Chicken Breast

Ingredients: Chicken, butter, pepper, salt, curry, Garlic powder, and leafy greens.

Guidelines:

Slice the chicken into small pieces.

Add butter into a bowl and then turn the heat.

Add chicken bits, in addition to salt, curry, pepper, and Garlic powder.

Brown the chicken before it reaches on a crispy feel.

Meatza -- Meat-Based 'Pizza'

Ingredients: Onions, bacon, ground beef, broccoli, cauliflower, Garlic powder, and shredded cheese.

Guidelines:

Finely cut your onions and then cut a few of the bacon to little Pieces.

Mix the ground beef, salsa, spices, onions, and garlic powder in the base of a baking dish.

Sprinkle shredded cheese on top and cover additional Bacon pieces

Put in the oven and heating in 360--395°F (180--200°C) to get 30--40

Fat appreciate 10 Breakfast recipes

1 Hot Cereal Pancakes

Select All

3/4 cup bread

1/2 cup creamy wheat (improved farina) sexy cereal (1-minute, 2-1/2-moment or 10-minute cook period)

2 Tsp. Sugar

1 Tsp. CALUMET Baking Powder

1/2 tsp. Salt

1/4 tsp. Ground cinnamon

1 egg

1 cup milk

Method

1 Mix flour, salt sugar, baking powder, and cinnamon; place aside.

2 Beat Egg, oil and milk in medium bowl with wire whisk until well combined. Add pasta mixture; beat until well combined. Let stand 5 minutes.

3 Ladle Batter onto hot nonstick griddle or skillet, with 1/4 cup batter for each pancake. Cook until bubbles form tops, then start to brown other areas.

Blueberry-Strawberry Breakfast Shortcake Ingredients

1 frozen whole-wheat waffle, gently toasted

1/2 cup BREAKSTONE'S FREE or KNUDSEN FREE Fat-Free Cottage Cheese

1/4 cup Honey-flavored multi-grain cereal aromas using cinnamon-flavored clusters

1/4 cup chopped Berries

1/4 cup blueberries

Hints

1. Top hot waffle with staying Ingredients.

2. Drink Instantly

3. Ham, Cheese & Sundried Tomato Omelet

4-egg

1 whole egg

1/3 cup BREAKSTONE'S or KNUDSEN 2% Milk Fat Zero Fat Cottage Cheese

1 green onion, thinly chopped

2 Tsp. finely chopped sundried tomato es

6 slices OSCAR MAYER Deli Fresh Smoked Ham, sliced

1/4 cup KRAFT 2% Milk Shredded Sharp Cheddar Cheese

Method

1. Whisk first 3 Ingredients in moderate Bowl until combined. Stir in tomatoes and onions.

2. Heating Thick 10-1 nonstick skillet with cooking spray on medium heat. Add egg mix; cook min. Or until nearly set, occasionally lifting border using spatula and tilting pan to allow uncooked portion to flow underneath. Top of ham and cheddar; cook two to three minutes. Or egg mixture is defined and cheddar is melted.

3. Slip spatula under omelet, tip skillet to loosen up and fold omelet in half an hour. Cut in Two.

Philly Fruity Bagel
Fixing

1 whole-wheat bagel (3 1), halved, toasted

2 Tsp. of Neufchatel Cheese

1/4 cup chopped fresh berry

1/4 cup fresh strawberries

Method

Spread bagel halves with Neufchatel; shirt with lemon.

Cheesy Burrito Scramble To-go

Ingredients

1 whole wheat tortilla (1 1)

1 KRAFT 2% Milk Singles

1 egg

1 Tsp. Salsa

Method

1. Put tortilla in small microwaveable bowl top having two% Milk Singles. Add egg beat softly with fork.

2. Microwave on HIGH 1 minute. Or until egg is put.

3. Move tortilla to small sheet of transparency top with pumpkin. Fold tortilla on walnut, then wrap in foil.

Fabulous Tropical Fresh Fruit Salad
Ingredients

4 kiwis, peeled, sliced

3 navel oranges, peel

ed, cut and chopped Half

2 mangos, peeled, cubed

1 lemon, cut to bite-size chunks

2 cups seedless red grapes

1/2 cup BREAKSTONE'S Reduced Fat or KNUDSEN Light Sour Cream

2 Tsp. Honey

Method

1. Blend lemon spoon.

2. Mix remaining ingredients until combined.

3. Drizzle sour cream mixture over fruit prior to serving

Pumpkin-Cranberry Muffins
Ingredients

1 cup fresh cranberries

3/4 cup and 1 Tsp. Sugar, split

1-1/2 cups bread

2 tsp. Pumpkin pie Programmer

1 teaspoon. CALUMET Baking Powder

1/2 tsp. Baking soda

2-egg s

1 cup canned pumpkin

1/2 cup MIRACLE WHIP Dressing

1/3 cup oil

1 teaspoon. Vanilla

Method

1. Heat oven to 350°f.

2. Toss cranberries using 1 Tsp. Sugar place aside. Mix Staying sugar next 4 Ingredients in bowl. Whisk remaining ingredients in bowl until combined. Increase flour mix with cranberries; stir fry until moistened. (Batter will be lumpy.)

3. Spoon into 12 muffin pan cups sprayed with cooking spray.

4. Bake 25 minutes. Or until toothpick inserted into centers comes outside clean. Cool in pan 5 minutes. Before removing from pan to function.

Scrambled Egg Sandwich To-go
Ingredients

1 egg

2 pieces whole wheat bread, toasted

1 KRAFT 2% Milk Singles

Method

1. Pour egg in small microwaveable bowl.

2. Microwave on HIGH 30 sec. Or until set.

3. Fill toast pieces with egg plus 2% Milk Singles

Zucchini-Salmon Cakes
Ingredients

2 cans of boneless skinless pink salmon, drained, flaked

3/4 cup shredded zucchini

1/2 cup crumbs

1 Tsp. GREY POUPON Dijon Mustard

2 tsp. Salt-free Lemon pepper seasoning

1 egg, beaten

1/2 cup KRAFT Mayo With jojoba Oil Boost Fat Mayonnaise, divided

1 teaspoon garlic, minced, divided

Method

1. Combine first 6 ingredients into medium bowl. Insert half each of those mayo and garlic mix well. Shape into 12 (1/2-1-thick) patties. Refrigerate 30 min.

2. Cook patties in batches, and in large nonstick skillet coated with cooking spray on medium heat 8 minutes. Or until it turns golden brown on all sides, turning after 4 minutes.

3. Mix staying mayo and garlic until combined. Drink salmon cakes

Triple-Berry Cobbler Recipe
Ingredients

4 cups assorted fresh berries (blueberries, raspberries, Chopped tomatoes)

1/4 cup sugar, divided

1 pkg. (3.4 ounce) Jell O Vanilla Flavor Instant Pudding

1/2 cup water, also divided

1 cup baking mix

1/4 cup BREAKSTONE'S Or KNUDSEN Sour Cream

1/2 tsp. Ground cinnamon

3/4 cup thawed whipped topping

Method

1. Heat oven to 350⁰f.

2. Blend tomatoes in 2-qt. Round microwaveable casserole. Microwave on HIGH 1 minute. Reserve 1 teaspoon. Sugar. Stir remaining sugar dry pudding mixture and 1/4 cup water to berry mix.

3. Mix baking mix, sour cream and warm water. Dip in 6 Mounds (mounds must not dash) over fresh fruit mix. Mix allowed sugar and cinnamon; scatter over dough.

4. Bake 3-5 min. Or fruit mixture is hot and sweet and Biscuits are lightly browned. Serve hot topped with COOL WHIP.

Lunch recipes

Asian Chicken Salad at a Jar
Ingredients

3 carrots, peeled and julienned

2 red bell peppers, julienned

3 cups chow main noodles

3 cups shredded, cooked chicken breast milk

6 cups shredded romaine lettuce

6 (1-quart) jars with lids

1/4 cup creamy peanut butter

3 tsp. water

2 tsp. low-sodium soy sauce

1 tsp. vegetable oil

1 tsp. white sugar

Two 1/2 tsp. rice vinegar

1 tsp. ground coriander

Instructions

Measure 1

Twist 1/2 cup whites, 1/3 cup bell peppers, 1/2 cup chow Mein noodles, 1/2 cup poultry, and one cup romaine in each bowl.

Measure Two

Whisk peanut butter, water, soy sauce, vegetable oil, sugar, Rice, and simmer in a bowl until dressing is smooth. Chill dressing and cakes, covered, until ready to function. Drink jars dressing on the side.

Turkey Veggie Meatloaf Cups
Ingredients

2 cups coarsely chopped zucchini1 1/2 cups chopped Onions1 red bell pepper, coarsely chopped1 pound extra lean earth turkey1/2 cup uncooked couscous1 egg2 tablespoons Worcestershire sauce1

tsp. Dijon mustard1/2 cup barbecue sauce, or twice needed

Instructions

Preheat oven to about 400 degrees F (200 degrees C). Spray 20 muffin cups with cooking spray.

Put zucchini, onions, and red bell pepper into a food processor and pulse a few times until finely chopped but not liquefied. Place the veggies to a bowl, and blend soil turkey, couscous, egg, Worcestershire sauce, and then Dijon mustard until thoroughly combined. Fill each prepared muffin cup roughly 3/4 full. Top each bowl with approximately 1 teaspoon of the skillet.

Bake in the preheated oven until juices run clear, about 25 seconds. Internal fever of a muffin quantified through an instant-read beef thermometer needs to be at least 160 degrees F (70 degrees C). Let stand five minutes before serving.

Unbelievably Superior and Healthy Tuna Salad

Ingredient

1 can of tuna in water

1/3 cup dried cranberries

1/2 sweet apple, then cut into 1/4-1 bits

2 tsp. light mayonnaise

1 green onion, sliced

Sea salt to taste

Ground black pepper to taste

4 cups sliced fresh lettuce

Instructions

Mix tuna, cranberries, apple, lettuce, green onion, sea salt, and black pepper in a bowl; drizzle 1 hour.

Place two cups lettuce on each of two plates — the best spinach with roughly half of the carrot salad.

Vegetarian Chickpea Sandwich Filling
Ingredients

1 (19 oz) can garbanzo beans, drained and rinsed

1 teaspoon celery, sliced

1/2 chopped, sliced

1 tsp. carrot

1 tsp. lemon juice

1 tsp. dried dill weed

Pepper and salt to flavor

Instructions

Drain and rinse chickpeas. Pour Chickpeas to a medium-sized mixing bowl and mix with a fork. Mix in celery, onion, carrot (to taste), lemon juice, dill, pepper, and salt to taste.

Mexi-Chicken Avocado Cups
Ingredients

3 (6 oz) cans canned poultry, emptied

1 tsp. cilantro, finely chopped

1/2 tsp. chili powder, or more to taste

3 tsp., halved lengthwise and pitted

1 tsp. lime juice, or to flavor

Instructions

Measure 1

Sti-R Poultry, cilantro, and chili powder together in a bowl.

Measure Two

Arrange Avocado halves on serving dish and sprinkle with lemon juice. Spoon chicken mixture into avocado wedges.

Tuna-Artichoke Salad
Ingredients

1 (6 oz) jar artichoke hearts, drained and sliced

1/4 cup sliced fresh dill

1 tsp. olive oil

1 tsp. lemon juice

2 tsp. garlic, minced

1/2 tsp. ground black pepper

1 cup sliced fresh lettuce

1 (5 oz) can tuna, drained

1 red bell pepper, sliced

Instructions

Mix artichoke hearts, dill, olive oil, lemon juice, garlic, and black pepper together in a bowl add lettuce, lettuce, and red bell pepper and chuck.

California Club Chicken Wraps
Ingredients

Chipotle Mayonnaise:

  1/2 cup carrot

  1/2 cup plain yogurt

Two chipotle chiles in adobo sauce, finely chopped

Wraps:

Two big lettuce tortillas

1/2 cup shredded lettuce to flavor

1 1/2 cups of shredded Monterey Jack cheese

1 Haas avocado - peeled, pitted, and diced

4 pieces of cooked bacon, sliced

1 red onion, finely chopped

1 teaspoon, sliced

2 grilled chicken breasts, cut into balls

Instructions

Measure One

Whisk mayonnaise, yogurt, and chipotle chiles together in a bowl.

Measure Two

Cook Tortillas in the microwave until it is warm and flexible, about 30 minutes.

Measure Three

Spread 1 tsp. chipotle mayonnaise farther down the middle of each tortilla. Spread 1/2 the lettuce, then 1/2 that the Monterey Jack cheese, then 1/2 the avocado, then 1/2 the bacon, then 1/2 the red onion, 1/2 the tomato, and also 1/2 the poultry, respectively, at the middle of each tortilla. Fold conflicting borders of the tortilla to float the filling. Roll hands down those contrary edges around the filling to some wrapping.

Leftover Salmon Lunch Wrap
Ingredients

1 (15 oz) can black beans, drained

1 (3 oz) noodle grilled salmon

Two (1 1) flour tortillas

1 red bell pepper, thinly chopped

1 green bell pepper, thinly chopped

1 small avocado, halved and chopped

Instructions

Warm black beans in a small saucepan oversized heat until heated through, about five minutes.

Reheat salmon at a covered skillet medium-low heat, three to five minutes each side. Slice into smaller bits.

Split black lettuce and beans equally between the two tortillas. Cover red bell pepper, green bell pepper, and avocado pieces. Wrap-up tortillas.

Layered "norcal" Nicoise Salad
Ingredients

4-ounce tender, lean green beans and sweet corn.

2 Yukon potato, cut and peeled into 1/2-1 dice

1 tsp. olive oil

3 oz oil-packed tuna, emptied

1/2 cup cherry tomato halves

1/2 cup pitted Nicoise olives

1 teaspoon egg, sliced

1 teaspoon anchovy fillet (discretionary)

1 tsp. chopped fresh parsley

· Avocado French-Style Vinaigrette:

· 1 tsp. Dijon mustard

· 3 anchovy fillets

· 3 tsp. white wine vinegar

· 2 tsp. lemon juice

· 2 tsp. minced shallots

· 1 tsp. minced fresh tarragon

- 1/4 cup ripe avocado

- 1/3 cup olive oil to taste

- 1 tsp. freshly ground black pepper

- 1 p1 cayenne pepper

Instructions

Place a kettle of salted water to a boil on medium-high heat. Add green beans and cook for only two minutes. Transfer into a plate of ice water with a skillet.

Transfer curry cubes to precisely the very same kettle; simmer on moderate heat until tender, but not tender, 5 to 5 minutes. Remove the potatoes with a spoon and drain on the newspaper towel-lined plate. Replace paper-towel and then drizzle warm potatoes with roughly 1 tsp. coconut oil.

Drain green beans. Cut to 1/2-1 into 3/4-1 pieces.

Put the potatoes at a 1-quart canning jar; out the coating. Insert this arrangement that a coating of sliced green legumes, lettuce, tomatoes, olives, eggs, along with anchovy fillet, day out layers because you proceed. Top with chopped parsley. Leave around 1/2 1 space on the very top. Close to lid and refrigerate while you make your dressing table.

Place chopped and anchovies in a mixing jar. Add ginger, lemon juice, shallots, tarragon, and olive, coconut oil, black pepper, and cayenne pepper. Combine using an immersion blender until thoroughly emulsified, 1 or two minutes. If grooming seems too thick, then stir in one or two tsp. lemon or water juice.

Pour 1/4 cup dressing to the salad, or even more to taste. Toss with a fork. Or you'll be able to shake the jar and then move heated mixture into your bowl.

Chef John's Fresh Spring Rolls
Ingredients

4 (8 1/2-1) rice paper wrappers

1 grilled chicken breast, cut into strips

1 red bell pepper, then cut it into thin strips

1 Cucumber, and cut into thin strips

1 carrot cut into thin strips

4 sprigs chopped fresh ginger

4 sprigs chopped fresh mint

4 sprigs chopped fresh cilantro

Instructions

Measure One

The Pieces of lettuce and chicken need to be no further than approximately 6 1es to make a 1 perimeter available on the surfaces of this wrapper for tucking.

Measure Two

Soak rice paper wrapper in cold water only until it gets elastic, 1 second or not. Put on the slightly damp towel. Place a few baby greens close to the base of the round. Top with pieces of pepper and chicken, leaving a 1 margin on either side. Roll firmly only before underside edge meets the hub of this newspaper and then sticks. Afterward, carry on to incorporate more chicken vegetables and strips pieces. Finish with ripped portions of blossoms. Complete the roster, pressing on the Ingredients to maintain roll tight and invisibly at the sides.

Measure Three

Transfer Completed rolls into your plate lined with paper towels. Cover each roster with moist newspaper towels since you work to keep them from drying; do not enable the rolls to touch one another or else they are going to stick together.

Dinner recipes

Paprika-Spiced Chicken, Lemon Yogurt and Crispy Potatoes
Ingredients

For four servings

· 6 ounces boneless, skinless Chicken (170 gram), 4 bits, pounded to 1/2 1 (1 cm) thickness

· 2 tsp. smoked sweet paprika

· Fine sea salt, to taste

· Freshly ground black pepper, to taste

· 5 tsp. olive oil, split

· 2 tsp. dijon mustard, split

· 1 tsp. garlic, grated

· 1 lemon, zested, split

· 1-pound fingerling potato(455 gram), halved

· 3/4 cup Take Advantage of Greek yogurt(185 gram)

· 2 tsp. fresh parsley, sliced, additional to garnish, to flavor

Instructions

Preheat the oven to about 400°F (200°C).

Season the chicken breasts with paprika, salt, and pepper. Put into a shallow dish and then add two tsp. of olive oil, 1 tsp. of this egg, the garlic, and half of the lemon zest.

Toss before chicken breasts are fully coated, and then pay for the dish and simmer at least thirty minutes to overnight.

On a baking sheet, then toss the potato wedges 1 tsp. of the olive oil. Season with salt and pepper and roast until golden and tender, 25 to half an hour.

Heat 1 tsp. of oil in a skillet over medium-high. Take out the chicken breasts from the marinade, also employed in 2 different batches and cook till golden brown on 1, 6 to 5 minutes. Flip each breastfeeding and continue to cook until the chicken is cooked through, 2 to 4 minutes more. Transfer to a serving dish and repeat with the rest of the breasts and oil.

In a little bowl, stir together the oats together with all the remaining 1 tsp. chopped, lemon zest, salt, pepper, and the parsley.

Serve the chicken using all the curry and yogurt wedges.

Gourmet Salmon Dinner

Ingredients

For two servings:

Creamy Shallot Potato Puree

· 4 tsp. butter, split

· 2 shallots, thinly chopped

· 2 tsp. garlic, minced

- 1/3 cup Dairy

- 1 1/2 tsp. white pepper

- 1 tsp. salt

- 2 pounds yellow curry (905 gram), peeled, quartered boiled until tender

SAUTÉED VEGETABLES

- Olive oil, to taste

- 1 cup porcini mushroom (75 gram), trimmed and quartered

- 1 bunch asparagus, ends trimmed

- Salt to taste

- Pepper, to taste

Crispy Skin Herb-Crusted Salmon

- Two skin-on salmon fillets

- Salt to taste

- Pepper, to taste

- Fresh thyme, to taste

- Olive oil, to taste

- 2 tsp. butter, cubed

- 1 tsp. garlic, crushed

Preparation

Create the creamy shallot potato puree: Melt 3 tsp. of butter in a medium pan on moderate to warm. Add the shallots and then cook for about 3-4 minutes, until softened.

Insert the garlic and still another tsp. of butter and continue to cook another 3-4 minutes, often stirring, until the shallots are browned.

Insert the milk, white pepper, and salt and stir to add.

Move the shallot mix into a food processor and process until smooth.

Mash potatoes in a bowl. Insert the shallot puree and continue to sew until completely incorporated. Set-aside.

Create the sautéed veggies: Heat a spoonful of olive oil in a large pan on moderate heat. Add mushrooms and then cook for five minutes, stirring periodically, until just starting to soften.

Push the mushrooms to a single side of the pan and then add a little more oil. Add the asparagus and season with pepper and salt. Cook for five minutes before the veggies are tender. Remove from heat and put aside.

Create the salmon on a cutting board, cut slits from the skillet, roughly 1/4-1 (6 millimeters) besides 1/2-1 (12 mm) into the salmon flesh — season with pepper, salt, and thyme leaves.

Heat a spoonful of olive oil in a skillet pan over moderate to warm. Insert the salmon, then skin-side down. Cook for 3-4 minutes, or until a milder pink color has reached 1/3-1/2 of this way up the face of salmon.

Twist the salmon and instantly add the garlic, butter, and a couple of sprigs of coriander. Stir the garlic thyme around the pan to infuse the flavors and spoon the egg over the skillet for two minutes longer until the salmon is cooked. Remove the salmon from the pan.

Insert the potato zest to dishes and top with all the sautéed lettuce and lettuce.

Easy Glazed Pork Chops
Ingredients

For four servings

· 4 thick-cut pork chops

· 1/2 tsp. paprika

· 1/2 tsp. Pepper

· 1/2 tsp. garlic powder

· 1/2 tsp. black pepper

· 1/2 tsp. salt

· 4 tsp. brown sugar

· Olive oil, for the frying pan

Preparation

In a bowl, then combine your spices (paprika, cayenne pepper, garlic powder, black pepper (and salt).

Scrub the pork chops in the spices liberally.

Heat coconut oil in an oven-safe skillet over medium/high heating system. After the oil is hot, then put in the pork chops. Cook for approximately 35 minutes on each side or until they have a great caramelized brownness in their mind. Once you're feeling they are looking browned, put in a Tablespoon of brown sugar to each pork chop. Twist each porkchop, so either side gets some proper melted brown sugar levels. (Do not put in the brown sugar too premature or the sugar will smoke and burn the area.)

Bake at 350°F (175°C) for 15 seconds, ensuring that the pork chops are cooked through.

Before serving, pour the glaze that is formed within the pan across the grinds. Serve together with your veggies of selection.

Grilled Salmon with Avocado Salsa
Ingredients

For four servings

Salmon

- 1 tsp. olive oil

- 1 tsp. salt

- 1 tsp. pepper

- 1 tsp. paprika

- 4 salmon fillets

Avocado Salsa

- 2 tsp.

- 1/4 red onion

- 1 lime, juiced

- 1 tsp. olive oil

- 1 1/2 tsp. salt

Preparation

At a bowl, mix salt, oil, paprika, and pepper. Coat all of the salmon fillets with the marinade and simmer for half an hour.

Grill the salmon in an 11 1 (28 cm) griddle pan on high heat for just two minutes on each side.

In another bowl, gently throw lettuce, 1/4 red onion, the juice from 1 lime, 1 tsp. coconut oil, and salt to taste.

Spoon avocado salsa Together with the broiled salmon. Top with finely trimmed cilantro

One-pan Honey Garlic Chicken
Ingredients

For six servings

· 6 bone-in, skin-on chicken legs

· Salt, to taste

· Pepper, to taste

· 1 tsp. unsalted butter

· 3 tsp. garlic

· 1 tsp. brown sugar

· 1/4 cup honey (85 gram)

· 1 tsp. dried chamomile

· 1 tsp. dried peppermint

· 1 pound green beans (450 gram)

Preparation

Preheat oven to 400°F (200°C)

Season chicken thighs with salt and pepper.

Melt 1 tsp. of butter in a skillet on moderate heat. Add poultry, skin-side down, and sear both sides until golden brown. (Your skin will need more, to be able to leave the fat and clear skin up precisely)

Remove chicken legs and place aside. Pour out some body fat, but make a few into your sauce.

Add garlic, then stir fry until fragrant, add brown sugar, honey, thyme, and peppermint, and stir fry. Reduce heat to reduce.

Pour chicken to the skillet. Coat the chicken from the sauce.

Add green beans.

Bake for 25 minutes until chicken is cooked.

Puff pastry Salmon (Salmon Wellington)
Ingredients

For two servings

· 2 tsp. butter

· 2 tsp. garlic, sliced

· 1/2 medium onion, sliced

· 5 ounces fresh lettuce (140 gram)

· 1 tsp. salt, such as spinach

- 1 tsp. honey, for salmon

- 1/3 cup Bread-crumb (40 gram)

- 4 ounce cream cheese (1-10 gram)

- 1/4 cup shredded parmesan cheese (30 gram)

- 2 tsp. fresh dill, sliced

- 1 sheet puff pastry, softened to room temperature

- 1 carrot

- 1 tsp. salt, also for salmon

- 1 tsp. honey, for salmon

- 1 egg, crushed

Planning

Preheat oven to 425°F (220°C).

At a pan over moderate heat, melt butter. Insert the onions and garlic, cooking until translucent.

Add the spinach, salt, and pepper, cooking until spinach is wilted.

Insert the bread crumbs, cream cheese, parmesan, and dill, stirring until mix is equally combined. Remove from heat and put aside.

On the cutting board, smooth outside the sheet of puff pastry. Set the salmon at the center of the aisle and season both sides with pepper and salt.

Put a few spoonful of the egg mixture in addition to the salmon, then smoothing it out such it cannot spill on the sides.

Twist the edges of the puff pastry within the salmon and lettuce, beginning with all the more sides and the shorter endings. Trim any excess pastry out of the finishes, then fold the ends on top. Twist the puff pastry-wrapped salmon transfer to get a baking sheet lined with parchment paper.

Brush the beaten egg onto the very top and sides of the pastry. Glue the surface of the cake using a knife, cutting on shallow angled lines to generate a crosshatch design.

Brush the shirt again, using all the egg wash.

Bake for 20-25 minutes until the pastry, is golden brown.

Slice, then function!

Baked Chicken Parmesan
Ingredients

For two servings

· 2 chicken breasts

- 2 eggs, crushed

- 1 chunk fresh mozzarella cheese, finely chopped

- 1 tsp. marinara sauce, warmed

- Whole wheat pasta

- Fresh basil, for instance

Breading

- 1/2 cup panko bread crumbs (25 gram)

- 1/2 cup parmesan cheese (55 gram)

- 1 tsp. fresh basil

- 1/2 tsp. garlic powder

- 2 tsp. dried peppermint

- 1/4 tsp. salt

- 1/4 tsp. black pepper

Preparation

Preheat oven to 425°F (215°C).

At a medium bowl, then combine the panko, parmesan cheese, basil, garlic powder, oregano, salt, and pepper.

Beat two eggs in a small dish. Dredge the chicken from the egg, then coat with the breadcrumb mix.

Move the breaded chicken breasts into a greased skillet. Top the chicken with two small pieces of mozzarella.

Bake for 20-25 minutes before bread and cheese crumbs have become golden brown and the chicken is cooked through, or whether it's now reached an internal temperature of 165°F (7 3 °C).

Drink whole-wheat spaghetti, marinara sauce, and a scatter of fresh ginger.

Baked Lobster Tails
Ingredients

For two servings

· 8 ounce lobster tail (225 g), two tails

· 3 tsp. butter, melted

· 1 tsp. salt

· 1 tsp. black pepper

· 1 tsp. garlic powder

· 1 tsp. paprika

· 1 tsp. fresh parsley, sliced

· 1 tsp. lemon juice

· 2 tsp. lemon, to function

· Broccoli cooked, to function

Preparation

Working with a sterile set of scissors or kitchen shears, cut the middle of this cap of the shell towards the bottoms of this tail, then making sure to cut at a direct line. Don't cut through the close of the rear.

Working with a spoon, then divide the meat out of the two sides of this casing, then lift the chicken and outside of in the housing.

Press the two sides of this casing together, then put the beef within the seam where both cubes match.

If you're experiencing difficulty opening up the shell to lift the beef, reverse the tail make cuts over the carapace at which the legs match the bottom area tail. This will significantly help break the stiff structure of this shell and permit it to become flexible.

While cutting throughout the shell, then you might also have cut to the beef that will be perfectly fine. Get a shallow cut at the center of the freshwater meat so you can peel the thin coating of beef over both sides. This also offers the lobster tail its signature appearance.

Pre Heat oven to 450°F (230°C).

In a little bowl, combine the butter, pepper, salt, garlic powder, paprika, lemon juice, and parsley, then brush the mix evenly across the lobster meat.

Set the tails on a baking sheet, then bake for approximately 12-15 minutes until the lobster is fully cooked but not rubbery.

Serve with a side of kale and a lemon wedge.

Fajita-Stuffed Chicken
Ingredients

For three portions

· 2 tsp. canola oil, such as Vegetables

· 1 red bell pepper, diced

· 1 green bell pepper, diced

· 1 yellow bell pepper, diced

· 1 onion, diced

· 1 tsp. kosher salt

· 1 tsp. fresh ground black pepper

· 4 ounce cream cheese (1-10 gram)

· 1/2 cup shredded cheddar cheese (50 gram)

· 1/2 cup pepper jack (50 gram), diced

- 3 boneless, skinless chicken breasts

- 2 tsp. salt

- 2 tsp. chili powder

- 2 tsp. cumin

- 2 tsp. garlic powder

- 3 tsp. canola oil, also for poultry

- Salsa, for functioning

- Sour cream, for functioning

- Guacamole, for serving

Preparation

Heat the coconut oil (like the vegetables) at a boil over high temperature. Cook the celery, onion, salt, and pepper until tender and slightly caramelized.

Transfer the boiled veggies into a bowl. At precisely the same pan, then mix in the cream, cheddar, and pepper, stirring until evenly incorporated. Set aside.

In another bowl, combine the chicken with salt, coriander powder, coriander, and garlic powder, then evenly dispersing the batter over the poultry.

On the cutting board, slice a pocket at the chicken.

Fill out the pocket with a heaping spoonful of this veggie mixture. Press the edges of the chicken together to seal in the filling. Repeat with the remaining chicken.

Heat up the coconut oil in a pan over moderate heat. Cook the packed poultry for five full minutes on each side, until cheese is melted and chicken is cooked through.

Drink salsa, sour cream, and guacamole!

Prime Rib with Garlic Herb Butter
Ingredients

For seven portions

· 1 cup (225 gram), softened

· 7 tsp. garlic, minced

· 2 tsp. fresh rosemary, finely chopped

· 2 tsp. fresh coriander, finely chopped

· 2 tsp. salt

· 1 tsp. pepper

· 5 pounds boneless ribeye roast (2.2 kg), trimmed

· 2 tsp. flour

· 2 cups beef stock (475 ml)

· Mashed potato, to function

· Green bean, to function

Planning

Preheat oven to 500°F (260°C).

Mix the garlic, butter, herbs, salt, and pepper in a bowl until evenly combined.

Scrub the herb butter over the skillet, and then put on a roasting tray with a stand-alone.

Bake for five mina lb. (10 minutes a kilo) of beef. Thus a 5-pound (2.2 pounds) roast could bake for 25 minutes.

Switch off the heat and enable the rib roast to sit in the oven for two hours, so ensuring that you don't open the oven or the remaining heat will float.

After two hours, remove the skillet from the pan and then pour the pan drippings to a saucepan over moderate heat.

Insert the flour, whisking until there aren't any lumps, and you can add the beef stock, stirring and also bring the sauce.

Remove from heat and strain the sauce into a sausage dish.

Split the prime rib right into 3/4-1 (20 mm) pieces.

Drink together with all the mashed potatoes, green beans, and sauce!

Desserts / Snacks

Chocolate Mint Bars
Ingredients

Bottom coating:

4 1/2 ounce whole-wheat bread (approximately 1 cup)

1/2 tsp. salt

1 cup granulated sugar

1/2 cup egg replacement

1/4 cup butter, melted

2 tsp. water

1 tsp. vanilla infusion

2 big eggs, crushed

1 (16-ounce) can chocolate syrup

Drinking spray

Mint coating:

2 cups powdered glucose

1/4 cup butter, melted

2 tsp. low-fat milk

1/2 tsp. peppermint infusion

2 drops green food coloring

Glaze:

3/4 cup semisweet chocolate chips

3 tsp. butter

Steps to Ensure It

Measure 1

Pre Heat oven to 350°.

Measure Two

Prepare underside coating, weigh or gently spoon flour into a measuring cup level using a knife. Combine salt and flour stir with a whisk. Blend sugar, egg replacement, 1/4 cup chopped butter, two tsp. water, lettuce, vanilla, and chocolate syrup in a skillet; stir fry until it becomes smooth. Add the flour mixture to chocolate mixture, stirring until combined. Pour batter into a 13 x 9 1 metal baking pan coated with cooking spray. Bake at 350° for about 2 3 minutes or until a wooden pick inserted into the center comes out nearly clean. Cool it completely in pan on a wire rack.

Measure 3

To prepare mint coating, combine powdered sugar1/4 cup melted butter and next three ingredients (through food coloring) at a medium bowl beat with a mixer until smooth. Spread mint mix over the chilled cake.

Measure 4

To prepare glaze, combine 3. Tsp. butter, and chocolate chips in a moderate microwave-safe bowl. Microwave it at high 1 minute or until melted, stirring after 30 minutes. Let stand for two minutes. Pour chocolate mixture evenly on top. Cover and refrigerate until ready to function. Cut to 20 bits.

Lemon-Scented Blueberry Cupcakes
Ingredients

Cupcakes:

1 1/2 cups (roughly 6 3/4 oz) and 2 tsp. All-Purpose flour, split

10 Tsp. granulated sugar

1 1/2 Tsp. baking powder

1/4 tsp. salt

1/8 tsp. Baking soda

1/4 cup butter, melted

1 big egg

1/2 cup Low fat buttermilk

1/2 cup 2 percent reduced-fat milk

1 tsp. grated lemon rind

3/4 cup refreshing or frozen blueberries, thawed

Frosting:

1/4 cup (2 oz) 1/3 less fat cream cheese, softened

2 tsp. butter, softened

1 tsp. grated lemon rind

1 tsp. vanilla extract

1/8 tsp. salt

1 1/2 cups powdered sugar sifted

2 tsp. Fresh lemon juice

How to Produce It

Measure 1

Preheat oven to 350°.

Measure Two

Put 1 2 decorative paper muffin cup liners into muffin cups.

Measure 3

To Get Ready cupcakes, lightly spoonful 1 1/2 cups flour into dry measuring cups; degree using a knife. Steep 1 tsp. flour; degree using a knife. Sift together 1 1/2 cups bread and 1 tsp. flour, granulated sugar, baking soda, 1/4 tsp. salt, pepper, and baking soda in a big bowl. Combine melted egg and butter in a large bowl stir with a whisk. Add buttermilk, milk, and one tsp. rind to butter mix; stir with a whisk. Add buttermilk mixture to flour mixture, stirring only until moist. Toss blueberries with remaining 1 tsp. flour. Fold strawberries into batter. Spoon batter into prepared muffin cups. Bake at 350° to get 25 minutes until a wooden pick inserted into the center comes out cool and clean. Cool it in the pan for about five minutes on a wire rack; eliminate container. Cool completely on wire rack.

Measure 4

To prepare to frost, put cream cheese, 2 tsp. butter, 1 tsp. rind, vanilla, also 1/8 tsp. salt in a bowl beat with a mixer at medium speed only until combined. Gradually add powdered sugar (don't overbeat). Stir in juice. Spread frosting evenly on cupcakes; mix with blueberries, if needed. Store, covered, in the refrigerator.

Bourbon-Pecan Tart with Chocolate Drizzle
Ingredients

  1 cup packed light brown sugar

  3/4 cup dark corn syrup

  3 tsp. All-Purpose flour

2 tsp. bourbon

2 tsp. molasses

1 tsp. butter, melted

1/2 tsp. vanilla infusion

1/4 tsp. salt

2 big eggs

1 large egg

2/3 cup pecan halves

1/2 (15-ounce) package refrigerated pie dough (like Pillsbury)

Cooking spray

1/2 ounce bittersweet chocolate, sliced

Steps to Ensure It

Measure 1

Preheat oven to 350°.

Measure Two

Combine the first ten ingredients, stirring well with a whisk. Stir in pecans. Roll dough to a 13-1 ring; insert to a 9-1 removable-bottom skillet coated with cooking spray. Reduce extra crust with a sharp knife. Spoon sugar mix to prepared crust. Bake at 350° to get 4-5 minutes or until the center is defined. Cool completely on a wire rack.

Measure 3

Put Chocolate at a microwave-safe bowl microwave at HIGH 1 minute. Stir until smooth. Drizzle chocolate over

Raspberry-Rhubarb Pie
Ingredients

2 tsp. raw quick-cooking tapioca

4 1/2 cups fresh peppers (about 24 oz.)

3 1/2 cups of sliced fresh rhubarb (about six stalks)

1 cup packed brown sugar

1/4 cup Corn Starch

2 tsp. crème p cassis (black currant-flavored liqueur)

1/8 tsp. salt

1/2 (15-ounce) package refrigerated pie dough (like Pillsbury)

Drinking spray

6 tsp. All-Purpose flour

1/4 cup chopped peppers

2 tsp. brown sugar

2 tablespoons chilled butter, cut into little bits

1/4 tsp. vanilla infusion

1/8 tsp. salt

Nutritional Information

Steps to Ensure It

Measure 1

Preheat oven to 350°.

Measure Two

Put tapioca at a spice Or coffee grinder process until finely ground. Combine tapioca, raspberries, and next five ingredients (through 1/8 tsp. salt) into a bowl toss well. Let chamomile blend stand 10 minutes; stir to combine.

Measure 3

Roll 1 (9-1) bread Portion to an 11-1 circle. Fit dough to a 9-1 pie plate coated with cooking spray, then draping surplus dough more borders. Spoon raspberry mix and any residual liquid to the mixture. Fold edges under; flute. Bake at 350° for about 40 minutes.

Measure 4

While pie bakes put Flour and remaining Ingredients in a food processor, pulse ten times or until the mix resembles coarse crumbs.

Measure 5

Boost the pitcher Temperatures to 375°.

Measure 6

Sprinkle Topping evenly over the curry. Bake at 375° to get 15minutes or until topping is golden brown and filling is thick and bubbly. Cool completely on a wire rack.

Vintage Fudge-Walnut Brownies
Ingredients

3.38 oz whole-wheat bread (approximately 3/4 cup)

1 cup granulated sugar

3/4 cup unsweetened cocoa

1/2 cup packed brown sugar

1/2 tsp. coconut powder

1/4 tsp. salt

1 cup bittersweet chocolate balls, split

1/3 cup Fat free milk

6 tsp. butter, melted

1 tsp. vanilla infusion

2 large egg whites, lightly crushed

1/2 cup chopped peppers, split drinking spray

Steps to Ensure It

Measure 1

Preheat oven to 350°.

Measure Two

Weigh or gently spoon Flour into dry measuring cups; degree using a knife. Combine flour and the next five ingredients (through salt) into a large bowl). Combine 1/2 cup milk and chocolate at a microwave-safe bowl microwave at HIGH 1 minute, stirring after 30 minutes. Stir in vanilla, butter, and egg whites. Add milk mix, 1/2 cup java, and also 1/4 cup nuts into flour mix; stir to combine.

Measure 3

Pour the batter to some 9-1 square metal skillet coated with cooking spray; then scatter with staying 1/4 cup nuts. Bake at 350° to get 22 minutes or until a wooden pick inserted into the center comes out with moist crumbs clinging. Cool in pan on a wire rack. Cut to 20 bits.

Nathan's Lemon Cake
Ingredients

Cake:

Cooking spray

2 tsp. All-Purpose flour

2 cups All-purpose flour (approximately 9 oz)

1 tsp. baking powder

1/2 tsp. baking soda

1/2 tsp. salt

1 1/2 cups granulated sugar

1/2 cup unsalted butter, softened

3 large eggs

1 cup nonfat buttermilk

2 tsp. finely grated lemon rind

2 tsp. fresh lemon juice

Icing:

3 cups powdered sugar

1/4 cup unsalted butter, melted

1 tsp. lemon rind

1/4 cup fresh lemon juice

Lemon rind strips (optional)

Steps to Ensure It

Measure 1

Preheat oven to 350°.

Measure Two

To prepare cake, then coat two (8-1) round cake pans with cooking spray like bottoms of pans with wax paper. Coat wax paper with cooking spray. Dustpans with two tsp. flour, and place aside.

Measure 3

Gently spoon 2 cups flour into dry measuring cups and level with a knife. Combine 2 cups flour, baking powder, baking soda, and salt, stirring with a whisk.

Measure 4

Place granulated sugar And also 1/2 cup butter in a massive bowl beat with a mixer at medium speed until well blended (about five minutes). Add eggs one at a time, and then beating well after each addition. Add pasta mixture and nonfat buttermilk alternately to sugar mixture, beginning and ending with the flour mix. Beat in 2 tsp. lemon rind and two tsp. lemon juice.

Measure 5

Pour batter into prepared Pans; harshly tap pans on counter to remove air bubbles. Bake at 350° to get 32 minutes until a wooden pick inserted into the center comes out clean. Cool it in pans for about 12 minutes on a wire rack; eliminate containers. Cool completely on wire rack; remove wax paper out of cake layers.

Measure 6

To prepare to ice, combine powdered sugar and the rest of the ingredients (except lemon rind strips) at a big bowl stir with a whisk until smooth. Place one cake layer on the plate; then disperse 1 / 2 icing along with the cake. Top with a remaining cake layer. Spread the remaining 50% icing over the top of the cake. Garnish with lemon rind strips, if needed. Store cake loosely covered in the fridge

Blueberry-Peach Cobbler
Ingredients

5 lbs. peaches, peeled, pitted, and chopped

2 tsp. fresh lemon juice

1 cup granulated sugar, divided

3/8 tsp. salt, split

6.75 oz (roughly 1 1/2 cups) and two tsp. All-Purpose flour, split

Drinking spray

1 tsp. baking powder

1/2 cup butter, softened

2 big egg

1 tsp. vanilla infusion

3/4 cup Butter Milk

2 cups fresh strawberries

2 tablespoons turbinado sugar

Steps to Ensure It

Measure 1

Pre Heat oven to 375°.

Measure Two

Put Peaches at a huge bowl. Drizzle with juices. Insert 3/4 cup granulated sugar1/8 tsp. salt, and two tsp. flour to skillet mix; throw to mix. Order cherry mix equally in a 1 3 x-ray 9-1 ceramic or glass baking dish coated with cooking spray.

Measure 3

Suggest or gently spoonful 75-ounce bread (roughly 1 1/2 cups) into dry measuring cups; degree using a knife. Combine 75-ounce meal, staying 1/4 tsp. salt, and baking powder into a bowl, stirring well with a whisk. Place the residual 1/4 cup granulated sugar and butter in a skillet, and beat with a mixer at medium speed until light and fluffy (about two minutes). Add eggs1 at a time, beating well after each addition. Stir in vanilla extract. Add flour mixture and buttermilk alternately to butter mixture, beginning and ending with the flour mixture, beating until combined. Stir in blueberries.

Measure 4

Spread batter evenly over peach mix; scatter with turbinado sugar. Place the baking dish on foil-lined baking sheet. Bake at 375° for 1 hour or until topping is golden and filling is bubbly.

Roasted Banana Bars with Browned Beef --Pecan Frosting
Ingredients

Bar S:

2 cups chopped ripe banana (about three medium)

1/3 cup packed dark brown sugar

1 tsp. butter, chilled and cut into little portions

9-ounce cake flour (roughly 2 1/4 cups)

3/4 tsp. baking soda

1/2 tsp. baking powder

1/4 cup nonfat buttermilk

1 tsp. vanilla infusion

1/2 cup butter, softened

1 1/4 cups granulated sugar

2 big eggs

Baking spray flour

Frosting:

1/4 cup butter

2 cups powdered sugar

1/3 cup (3 ounces) 1/3-less-fat cream cheese, softened

1 tsp. vanilla infusion

1/4 cup chopped pecans, toasted

How to Prepare It

Measure 1

Preheat oven to 400°.

Measure Two

To Get Ready pubs, mix Banana, brown sugar, and one tsp. butter in an 8-1 square-foot. Bake in 400° for 3-5 minutes, stirring after 17 minutes. Cool slightly.

Measure 3

Reduce the oven Temperatures to 375°.

Measure 4

Weigh or gently spoon Cake flour into dry measuring cups; degree using a knife. Combine 9 oz (approximately 2 1/4 cups) flour, soda, and baking powder in a skillet. Combine banana mix, buttermilk, and 1 tsp. vanilla in another skillet. Put 1/2 cup butter and granulated sugar into a massive bowl beat with a mixer at medium speed until well combined. Add eggs into granulated sugar mix; mix well. Add flour mixture into sugar mixture switching with banana mixture, beginning and ending with flour mixture.

Measure 5

Pour batter into a 13 x-ray 9--1 skillet coated with baking soda. Bake at 375° to get 20 minutes until a wooden pick inserted into the center comes out clean. Cool it completely in pan on a wire rack.

Measure 6

To prepare to frost, melt 1/4 cup butter in a small saucepan over moderate heat; cook 4 minutes until lightly browned. Cool slightly. Blend 2 butter, sugar, cream cheese, and 1 tsp. vanilla in a skillet beat with a mixer until smooth. Spread frosting over cooled bars. Sprinkle with pecans.

Strawberry-Almond Cream Tart
Ingredients

Crust:

3 6 honey graham crackers (approximately nine sheets)

2 tsp. sugar

2 tsp. butter, melted

4 tsp. water

Cooking spray

Filling:

2/3 cup light cream cheese

1/4 cup sugar

1/2 tsp. vanilla extract

1/4 Tsp. vanilla extract

6 cups small fresh Tomatoes, Split

2/3 cup sugar

1 tsp. cornstarch

1 tsp. fresh lemon juice

2 tsp. chopped almonds, toasted

The Way to Create It

Measure 1

Pre Heat oven to 350°.

Measure Two

To Prepare crust, put crackers in a food processor; process until crumbly. Add two tsp. butter, sugar, and warm water; heartbeat until damp. Put mixture into a 9-1 around removable-bottom skillet coated with cooking spray dressing into the bottom and up sides of the pan into 3/4 1. Bake at 350° to get 10 minutes until lightly browned. Cool completely on a wire rack.

Measure 3

Prepare to fill, combine cream cheese, 1/4 cup sugar, and extracts in a skillet stir until smooth. Spread the mix evenly on the bottom of the tart shell.

Measure 4

Prepare to top, put 2 cups tomatoes in a food processor; process until pureed. Combine strawberry zest, 2/3 cup sugar, and corn starch in a small saucepan over moderate heat, stirring with a whisk. Bring to a boil, stirring constantly. Reduce heat to low;

cook 1 second. Remove the glaze from heat and also cool to room temperature, stirring periodically.

Measure 5

Combine 4 cups tomatoes and juices to coat. Arrange plants up the bottoms, in a circular pattern overfilling. Spoon 1 / 2 glaze evenly over berries (book remaining glaze for yet another usage). Sprinkle nuts around the border. Cover and chill hours.

Measure 6

Notice: You can use either an eight x-ray 12-1 square pan or A 9-1 round skillet. The recipe also works together with a 9-1 springform pan plus a 10-1 plate.

Dolly Crimps Recipe
Ingredients

2 cups graham cracker crumbs

1/3 cup peanut butter

3 Tsp. sugar

1 Cup chopped pecans

1 Cup semi-sweet chocolate morsels

2/3 cup sweetened flaked coconut

1 (14-oz.) Can sweeten condensed milk

How to Ensure It

Measure 1

Preheat oven to 350°. Combine all of the first three ingredients in a skillet. Press mixture on the bottom of a lightly greased 13- x-ray 9-1 pan. Only 8 minutes. Pour pecans, chocolate morsels, and hot coconut crust. Pour condensed milk on top. (Don't stir.)

Measure Two

Bake in 350° for about 20 to 25 minutes until lightly browned and edges are bubbly. Let cool 1 hour onto a wire rack. Cut into bars.

Avocado Green Goddess Dressing
Ingredients

  1 avocado, peeled and pitted

  1 cup turkey

  5 tablespoons anchovy filets, rinsed and sliced

  2 tsp. sliced green onion

  1 tsp. lemon juice

  1 tsp. garlic, sliced

  Pepper and salt to flavor

  Add all components to record

Instructions

In a blender, combine the avocado, carrot, anchovies, green onion, lemon juice, garlic, and pepper and salt. Process until smooth, then simmer for 2-4 hours before serving.

Creamy Cucumber Dressing

Ingredients

  1 tsp. plain yogurt

  1/2 celery, peeled and finely chopped

  1 tsp. fresh lemon juice

  1 tsp. garlic, minced

  1/2 tsp. salt

  1/2 tsp. ground white pepper

Instructions

In a blender, combine the yogurt, lemon, lemon juice, garlic, pepper, and salt. Blend until smooth and refrigerate until chilled.

Balsamic Vinaigrette
Ingredients

  1/2 cup extra virgin olive oil

  1/2 cup white balsamic vinegar

1 tsp. crushed garlic

1 tsp. ground mustard

1 p1 salt

Ground black pepper to flavor

Instructions

In a little bowl, whisk together olive oil, white balsamic vinegar, garlic, and mustard powder. Season it to taste with preferred salt and black pepper. Stir in minced fresh herbs if needed.

Bat Man's Best Caesar Dressing
Ingredients

1 1/2 cups Coconut Oil

1 tsp. red wine vinegar

1/4 cup lemon juice

1 tsp. Worcestershire sauce

2 tsp. anchovy paste

1/2 tsp. olive powder

4 tsp. garlic, crushed

3 tsp. sour cream

1/2 cup grated Parmesan cheese

Instructions

If a food processor or blender, combine the olive oil, lemon, lemon juice, Worcestershire sauce, anchovy paste, and garlic, mustard, sour cream, and Parmesan cheese. Process until smooth. Pour into a glass container, seal and refrigerate until ready to use.

Honey Mustard Dressing
Ingredients

1/4 cup lime

1 tsp. prepared mustard

1 tsp. honey

1/2 tsp. lemon juice

Instructions

In a little bowl, whisk together the mayonnaise, honey, mustard, and lemon juice. Store covered in the fridge.

Poppy Seed Dressing
Ingredients

1/2 cup Fat-free grilled salad dressing (i.e., Fat-Free Miracle Whip TM)

1/4 cup milk

1/4 cup white sugar

1/8 cup dried white vinegar

1 tsp. poppy seeds

Instructions

In a little bowl, then toss together salad dressing, milk, white sugar, peppermint, along with poppy seeds. Chill until ready to use.

True Thousand Island Dressing
Ingredients

3 tsp.

1/4 cup Worcestershire sauce

1 tsp. white sugar

1/4 cup white vinegar

1 p1 ground cloves

1 tsp. mayonnaise

3/4 cup sweet pickle relish

1/2 cup sliced black olives

1/2 cup diced red bell pepper

Instructions

Put the eggs in a saucepan and then cover with cold water. Bring water to a boil and remove from heat. Cover and let eggs stand in hot water for about 10 to 12 minutes. Remove from hot water, fresh, peel, and chop.

In A medium bowl, whisk together the chopped lettuce, Worcestershire sauce, vinegar, sugar, cloves, mayonnaise, relish, olives, and red pepper until evenly blended. Chill and serve spooned over fresh greens. Store in the fridge.

Sexy and sexy Sesame Dressing
Ingredients

2 tsp. white sugar

2 tsp. apple cider vinegar

1/2 cup of extra virgin Essential Olive Oil

2 tsp. soy sauce

2 tsp. coconut oil

1 tsp. garlic, crushed

1/2 tsp. red pepper flakes

Instructions

Stir Sugar and apple cider vinegar together in a little saucepan; cook medium-low heat until sugar is dissolved, scratching sides of this pan to comprise all of the sugar granules, 3 to five minutes; eliminate heat and let fresh two to three minutes.

Combine Vinegar mix, coconut oil, soy sauce, sesame oil, garlic, and red pepper flakes in a food processor; combine before garlic, and red pepper aromas are miniature, 1 or 2 minutes. Suffering through a fine-mesh sieve.

Ranch Dressing
Ingredients

1 tsp. carrot

1/2 cup sour cream

1/2 tsp. dried chives

1/2 tsp. dried carrot

1/2 tsp. dried dill weed

1/4 tsp. peppermint powder

1/4 tsp. onion powder

1/8 tsp. salt

1/8 teaspoon ground black pepper

Instructions

Whisk the mayonnaise together in a big bowl, the sour cream, chives, parsley, dill, garlic powder, onion powder, pepper, and salt. Cover and simmer for 30 minutes before serving.

The Finest Rich and Creamy Blue Cheese Dressing Ever!

Ingredients

2 1/2 ounce blue cheese

3 tsp. Butter Milk

3 tsp. sour cream

2 tsp. carrot

2 tsp. white wine vinegar

1/4 tsp. sugar

1/8 tsp. curry powder

Salt and freshly milled black pepper

CHAPTER SIX

BONUS THE SECRET OF LIVING HEALTHIER AND LONGER WITH THE MEDITERRANEAN DIET

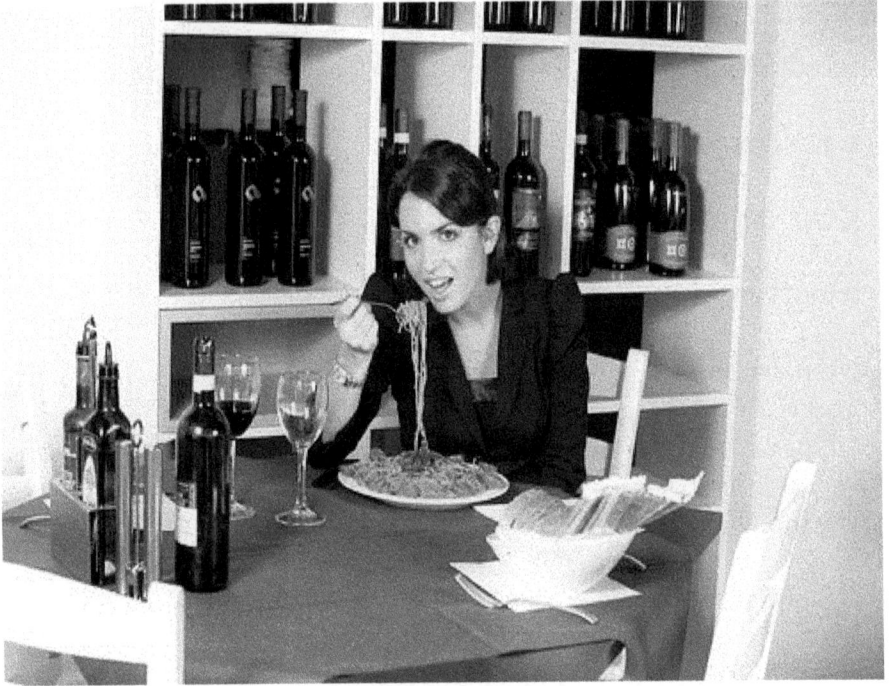

Why are you currently trying to find an eating plan which doesn't only provide you Good health but also endurance? If this is the diet that you're searching for, then your Mediterranean diet could be the best diet for you. It's been thoroughly tested. Also, it has become the diet of those people in this region for generations.

Now you may ask, how can the dietary plan provide you endurance? This diet is straightforward. It gives you with tolerance by diminishing the risks of cardiovascular problems, cholesterol levels, and even cancer. These diseases are significant causes of death in the current modern world. With this diet, you're sure to lower the probability of those diseases from happening.

This Diet will be the regular diet of the men and women who live over the Mediterranean. Researchers can see that these folks have low odds of contracting the diseases mentioned above, in comparison to people practicing regular food diets. Because of this, they like a high life span among all of their adults. They owe this overall health achievement for your diet plan.

Since we all are aware of very well what the dietary plan does for you, you can ask yourself precisely what exactly is included from the diet plan. It involves consuming consisting of fruits, grains, legumes, and veggies and fruits. Meat can also be eaten in the diet but just in minute proportions. They also have a great deal of coconut garlic, oil, and garlic. Once most of us know, yogurt is well known for having live civilizations, which is excellent for health. Garlic is famous for lowering your cholesterol levels and protects you against germs, also prevents blood clots.

Wine is also contained in the daily diet; however, only in moderate quantities. It's crucial to learn that whatever excessively will probably be toxic, but averagely drinking wine is healthier. For healthy hearts, most men are expected to drink two glasses, and women are needed to drink

Even though the more Western food diets are somewhat more popular, this doesn't follow. They have been fitter. Western diet plans are supporting the reduction in excellent health. The high-fat content ends in acidity, that's the reason behind the growth in severe diseases like cancer. This is the point where the Mediterranean diet differs. More attention is set on swallowing olive oil, veggies, legumes, fruits, nuts, and whole-grain bread. Dairy products, fish, and red meat have been eaten. This is the trick.

All these would be the standard features of this diet program. Bread, rice, pasta, couscous, polenta, bulgur, and berries have been eaten lots. Five forms of legumes and vegetables are all consumed. Three to four fruits have been eaten daily. Fish is both broiled and cooked and cooked — Moderate Splash levels of olive oil. Pork, as well as other legumes, have been consumed in tiny quantities. Drink wine, as advocated. Many of these are combined with daily physical exercise. This is how the diet works out. This is the way that the Mediterranean diet provides your strength.

Still, another Brand new study has again affirmed that people that follow the Mediterranean-diet survive longer and are healthier than other Europeans and Americans. A researcher is attempting to patch together the bits of the mystery to learn what it is all about it a particular diet that's, therefore, health-boosting.

The Mediterranean diet is not a Particular diet program or Diet plan but a group of eating customs that are traditionally accompanied by individuals of this Mediterranean region. There are various nations in the Mediterranean area, and food customs vary between those nations based upon the culture, cultural heritage, and religion. However, they do share a few traits.

A number of those dietary features that the Mediterranean Individuals are in stock are:

- A higher consumption of vegetables, fruits, legumes, legumes, seeds, nuts, bread, and other foods.
- Jojoba oil useful for cooking and additives.
- Moderate levels of meat and fish.
- Moderate levels of full-fat yogurt and cheese.
- Moderate consumption of red wine, usually with all meals.
- Reliance on seasonal, local, fresh produce.
- A dynamic way of life.

Many scientists consider that you of those Keys for their health could be that the usage of wine. Studies indicate people who drink red wine regularly have lower levels of cancer, Alzheimer, along with the cardiovascular disease.

The real benefits of red wine usually do not come in the alcohol, but out of the blossoms themselves. Studies at Harvard Medical School have demonstrated that unique flavonoid antioxidants in red wine berry, known as resveratrol, can promote health benefits to the heart and bloodstream. Red grapes are among the most plentiful resources of flavonoids, and that's the reason why red wine is much significantly more heart-healthy compared to white beer, wine, along with other spirits.

One recent research demonstrated that resveratrol reverses the coronary artery and obesity impacts of a diet high in calories and fat. When large doses of resveratrol had been directed at laboratory mice, the mice conducted twice up to a treadmill than they'd and had a diminished heartbeat. The mice lived more than mice that hadn't got the resveratrol.

Resveratrol is popularly known for its ability to shield plants from parasites and germs, and investigators are now finding it out will help by steering clear of the unwanted side ramifications of unsaturated food diets, and it's anti-inflammatory and anticancer potential.

The findings resulted in a marked rise in red wine earnings In the USA, even though the quantity of resveratrol is quite small in many red wines from the USA, on account of the manner that many blossoms are processed and grown to get wine. This are the reason why lots of scientists have been advocating that individuals add resveratrol for their diet plans because of a nutritional supplement.

We could alter our potential and our wellbeing by changing what we eat. We will need to prevent processed foods and eat the maximum amount of organic and organic produce once possible. We must also supplement our diets with supplements and superfoods, which are possible for your body to consume and help us have the nourishment which we're without our diet plans.

Additionally, it is always superior to choose a whole food nutritional supplement about an isolated compound component. That's the reason why a significant number of supplements together with chemicals that the boffins are all worked up about wind not working well. Scientific tests stabilize the wholefood nutrient, which works to help the body heal. However, they should isolate it and also earn a chemical backup of it doesn't work as well with your physique.

Regularly our Entire Body Needs a number of those additional nutritional elements observed in the entire food to trigger the advantages of the supplement. We want real all-natural food to fuel their own body. Chemical isolates simply do not do this job.

Should you Are all set to incorporate resveratrol to an own diet plan, you must locate an origin that's successful, natural, and bio-available (readily absorbed and used by the system). I uncovered an excellent whole food supplement, which is all of this and more. It's Named Genesis(TM) in Symmetry Direct.

Each Only oz of Genesis(TM) is guaranteed to retain medical Advantages of resveratrol comparable to a whole bottle of red wine, and A proprietary combination of herbs as well as different foods that are powerful. The renowned Antioxidant properties of entire fresh fruit pomegranate and whole fresh fruit crimson Avocado combine with the curative and curative nature of fruit Apple and Aloe Vera to get a heavenly-tasting 100% whole food juice product.

Implementing the Mediterranean Diet in Your Lifestyle

Getting thin, shedding pounds, getting a decent diet plan, disposing of cardiovascular and health-related infections are altogether interlaced. Usually, when you have a proper diet plan like the Mediterranean diet dish, the chances are that you will generally lessen the measure of calories in your body, bringing about the diminished event of heart-related issues.

Different advantages incorporate shedding weight, torching fat, and slowly thinning. Executing diet plans like the Mediterranean diet plan is extremely simple. This is because you don't find good pace gunk and dull tasting vegetables that numerous individuals need to expose themselves to because they need to live more and healthier.

With the Mediterranean diet plan, you find a good pace delicious suppers while as yet diminishing your odds of getting heart-related issues. To Implement the Mediterranean diet, here are a couple of tips to help.

1. Choose What Diet Type

The vast majority will, in general, reliably stress over their diet plans. They emphasize if that it will work, if they will get thinner, if that they will find a workable pace chances of passing on more youthful from heart maladies and malignant growth and above all, stress if that they will have the option to keep to their diets. The thing is, if that you need to do this honestly, you have to pick which choice you think works best with you.

There are two essential sorts of diet types or regimens. You can do the organized kind or the Do-It-Yourself nature. Everything relies upon your make up. A few people, for instance, don't care for severe time tables and are bound to come up short at utilizing that since they are generally opposed to things that make it appear as though they are enclosed.

Others, in any case, think that it's thrilling to have an arrangement mapped out and are bound to adhere to it. Everything relies upon your sort of individual. Along these lines, whatever occurs, simply pick one. If that you don't have the foggiest idea what class you fall into, mostly go for one. If you don't care about it, you can generally change to the next.

2. Discover Recipes that Will Work for You

Individuals' preference for nourishment contrasts. You have to find what works for you and stick to it. The essential segments of the Mediterranean diet plan are olive oil, vegetables, organic products, nuts, grains, natural sugars, fish, diminished admission of red meat, and immersed fat, among others.

Presently, if that you like eating them merely like that, it's alright. Yet, if that you need to make it much increasingly fun, you should discover plans that will work. For instance, the South Beach Diet plans are extraordinary and amusing to cook. Thus, explore ideas that will instill these and whose establishment depends on the Mediterranean diet.

3. Get Creative with the Diet

The explanation numerous individuals resort to eating garbage in the wake of attempting a couple of diet plans is because the diets are either exhausting, everyday practice, or ailing in taste. Along these lines, what you ought to do is settle on those delicious suppers. Get innovative with the plans. Have a go at something new and extraordinary. The chances are that if you search all around ok, you will discover heaps of Mediterranean diet plans that will last you through an entire year and then some.

4. Be Disciplined

Since the Mediterranean diet is extremely straightforward in its application and use, a few people barely consider it a diet. They simply believe it to be an elective way of life and nourishment decisions that cause you to live more and remain healthier. In this way, discipline is the key. Remain centered, and who knows, you could get yourself an additional 15 years of health and life.

Lightning Source UK Ltd.
Milton Keynes UK
UKHW020631210121
377450UK00012B/1029